LUPUS OR ME?

I Chose Me!

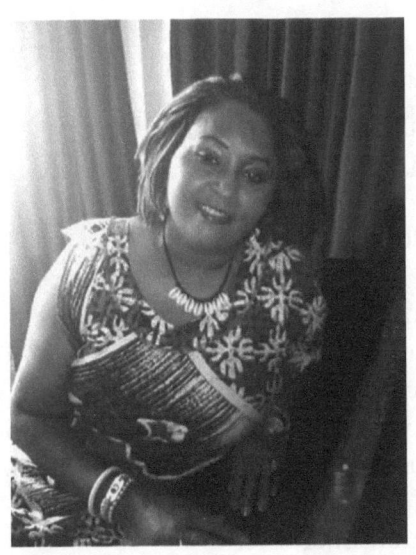

LOLA AFORO

ISBN 978-1-0980-3809-0 (paperback)
ISBN 978-1-0980-3810-6 (digital)

Christian Faith Publishing, Inc.
832 Park Avenue
Meadville, PA 16335
www.christianfaithpublishing.com

Printed in the United States of America

To all lupus sufferers and especially me. It is my hope to share my story and hope that people will enjoy my story, learn from it and be enlightened about lupus, as well as take care of you! Do not feel judged!

Contents

Introduction...7

Chapter 1: My Life before Lupus 9

Chapter 2: Diagnosis and Reactions............................25

Chapter 3: Battles 29

Chapter 4: Putting the Pieces of My Lupus Puzzle Together.......59

Chapter 5: Choosing Me!..71

Introduction

Lupus or Me? I Chose Me! This book is a project that I started writing in my mind in the late 1990s after I was diagnosed with lupus. I was diagnosed with lupus in 1998. As a young woman in my early thirties, I did not quite understand the illness. I know that it brought many changes in my life and I was ill many a time. I questioned it in my mind and every step of the way. In fact, I had to go on sick leave for the very first time in my work life in the summer of 1998. Then I started to realize that I have a serious situation at hand. At that time, I was a divorcee in my early thirties raising my daughter by myself. I have strong support from families and friends who helped me a great deal and they still continue to render support.

I decided to read and educate myself about lupus! I learned about many lupus stories, but it did not make sense to me still. I learned it is an immune disease, and it may affect organs in your body. At that point, I decided that lupus will never take over my life. I have fought many battles in my life and I have managed to win, lupus will not stop me. With this in mind, I geared up for the battle with lupus, and I was determined to win.

One major fact I learnt about lupus is that lupus sufferers must stay away from any stressful situations and environment. So I try to eliminate stressful events, situations, and environment in my life. Stresses dealing with my daughter and single mother life, families, and friends, I manage to the best of my ability. The stresses that were problematic, I off-loaded. Luckily, my daughter, friends, and family were cooperative and very understanding; which is a blessing with dealing with lupus.

This book will narrate my life before lupus and why I think that life brought on lupus and how I continue with the daily struggles with lupus. As the struggles continue, I vouched that I will win my battles with lupus and I will live to enjoy my daughter and family, who make life more beautiful each day. My families as well as my friends are my source of support and strength. I look forward to enjoying quality time with all these people and enjoy life as much as possible. Above all, I have learned to make God the driver of my life as I continue to strengthen my Catholicism faith. God is my foundation and my rock. I will praise his name each and every day. Because of this, I chose "Me" over lupus.

1

My Life before Lupus

I was born in Freetown, Sierra Leone, West Africa. I come from a polygamous family. My father had several wives and many children. Our mother, Mrs. Jemie Aforo, had six daughters and one son living. I am the fifth child. My parents worked hard to ensure that we went to school. My mother was the champion in this area. She worked tirelessly to ensure that her young ones went to school. She also helped educate many young people in the community. I attended both elementary and secondary schools in Freetown, the capital city of Sierra Leone.

As a young girl, I encountered countless physical, emotional, and sexual abuses and molestations from my relatives and people in the community. These abuses were never talked about by anyone. I thought it was normal to experience such abuses. I remembered seeing young girls going through similar experiences often. One particular case I recalled was an eight-year-old girl, who was sent to the market and ended up getting sexual abused by an older respectable man. It died out like breeze in the community. In fact, the poor girl was blamed for even entering the premises of the man. So as children, we dealt with sexual abuses silently and moved on. Because children are always blamed for the action.

During my high school years, I dated few young men. I liked some of them, and there was one I fell in love with, but he travelled out of the country to pursue his education. Hence, that became the end of our love story. In a way, I am thankful for the man I ended up with as through that relationship I am blessed with an unconditional love that I experienced with my daughter. My mother and I shared a bond of unconditional love, as well as my first love, but the bond I enjoy with my daughter is amazing.

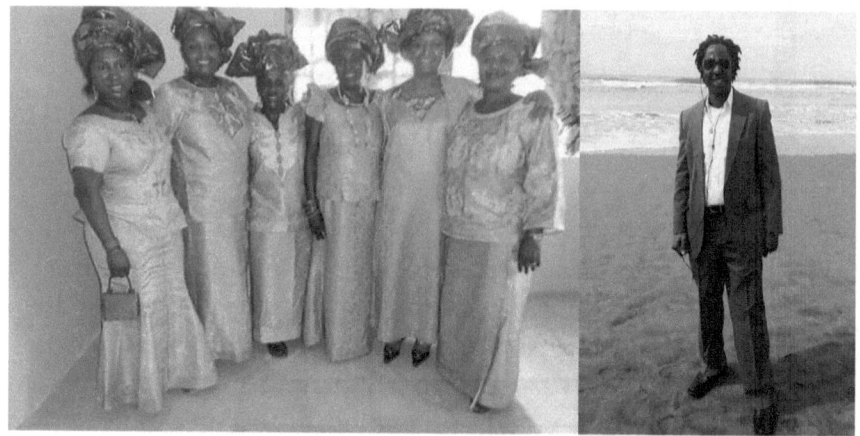

Me and my six sisters, L to R: The first born, Mrs. Ebun Strasser King; second, Mrs. Ade Lekoetje; third, Mrs. Feyi Akinbobolai; fourth, Ms. Remi Aforo; fifth, Ms. Lola Aforo; and sixth, Mrs. Comfort Foon. We have one brother, who is the last born and we call him PA.

During my high school years, I was initiated into the female genital mutilation (FGM) society. This usually takes place when young girls are almost finished with high school or approaching puberty. Their families, especially their mothers will introduce the idea. Girls usually have no choice or say-so on this matter. It was the most horrific experience in my youthful life. Up till now, it feels like it is very recent! That memory has never left me. However, I have been able to conquer this experience or leave it in the back burner of my mind while I move on in life. It is very common for young girls to be initiated into FGM so that upon graduation, you are accepted easily in your community and people tend to respect you more. It also prepares young girls for marriage. After FGM, most girls are married off. To say the least, FGM has left an everlasting scar in my life emotionally, mentally, and physically.

Anyhow, in my final year of high school I met someone, who later became my husband. He was studious and hardworking. My sisters and family knew him very well, and he was highly respected in the community. My sisters have great respect for him too. They were happy we were dating as well. We dated in Freetown for a while then he got a scholarship to further his studies in the United States. He wanted me to join him in the United States so we got married in June 1982.

My husband moved to the United States and filed the necessary documents for me to join him in the United States. At age eighteen on September 2, 1983, I left the shores of Sierra Leone, West Africa, to join him. He was located in Tallahassee, Florida, and he was a master's student at Florida State University. I was very excited to come to see the new world, where every young person from my part of the world aspires to come. I was eagerly looking forward even though I had mixed feelings. I flew on Sierra Leone Airways from Sierra Leone to London, England. I cried all the way to London and did not even eat in the plane. I was very sad as I was leaving my families along with my friends. But I was meeting my best friend, Abi B, in London so it made me a bit happy and gave me something to look forward to. I have not seen her in a very long time so the thoughts of seeing her again were exciting. I was so looking forward to our meeting that my flight to London was not so bad. Although I cried most of the way to London, I slept as well. Abi B met me at London Gatwick

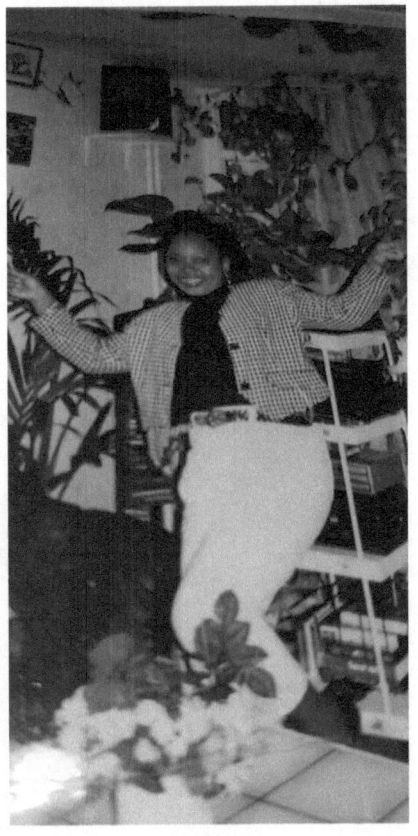

Abi B-BFF

Airport. It was great to see her! We hugged and cried when we met. It was very nice to see her and visited with her.

We both wished I had stayed in London for a few days, but my husband was against it. So I had to catch another flight to the USA right away. It was so sad to leave her again, but I know in due time, I will see her again. I flew on Air Jamaica directly to Miami, Florida. It was a very long flight compared to flying from Freetown to London. I arrived in Miami around 1:00 p.m. on September 3, 1983. Then I boarded another flight to Tallahassee, Florida. It has been a long and interesting journey. Miami's airport was big, and I almost got lost. The fact that I did not have anyone meeting me at a big airport like Miami's was traumatic for me. However, Tallahassee's airport was just right for a young West African girl, who was landing in the United States for the very first time. It was just a bit bigger than my airport, and I felt more at ease than at Miami Airport. I arrived around 7:00 p.m. on September 3, 1983, in Tallahassee. Felix met me at the airport. He came with a Caucasian lady to pick me up. He introduced her to me as Julie Goodwin. Since that night, Julie and I have become as the Americans would say "peas and carrots," inseparable. She has proved to be a friend, a mentor, and a sister till today.

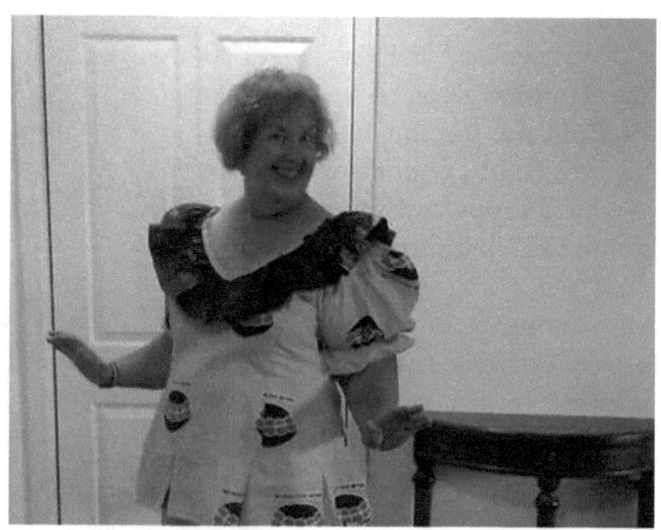

Dr. Julie Goodwin, mentor and friend

In Tallahassee, I was not sure of what life will be like! I was worried about foods, the weather, clothing, etc. Since it is a sub-tropical climate it is very similar to Freetown's climate. I found similar foods and clothing, which made me happy. It only gets a bit cold in January and February. Generally, the weather was favorable. Otherwise, Tallahassee was a pleasant change. It was easy to make friends as we lived in a student-centered housing environment with mostly international students. Additionally, I had nice African braids on my hair which attracted people toward me. The ladies and some men liked it and wanted their hair braided as well. Luckily for me, I could braid. So I quickly became famous for African hair braiding and soon started earning money from doing hair. My husband made pictures of my work and I started to generate clienteles right away. Through hair braiding, I met students from every continent. I also met a few other Sierra Leoneans as well. One Sierra Leone lady who was my age group became friends with me and we became much like sisters. We shared notes as well as encouraged each other over the years. One story that we shared was about our very first night with our husbands in Tallahassee. It was horrific! Our husbands left us behind in Sierra Leone to join them later. Apparently both our husbands heard stories that we cheated and had boyfriends in their absence. Instead of welcoming their wives with hugs, romance, and love, we were welcomed with physical abuse! That was a very cold night for me, and I wanted to return back to Sierra Leone badly. The road was far, and I wanted to be successful in America. Since it's an opportunity, I overlooked the physical abuse and emotional torment. This abuse continued for the most part of our marriage. There were about five other Sierra Leoneans and other Africans that I met in Tallahassee as well. We had international gatherings at least once a month with potluck dinners. It was fun. Julie, my friend, was always part of the gathering as she lived in the community with her two girls.

One area that was difficult for me to cope with in the United States was my experience with the health system. The first time Felix took me to a clinic, I had to be examined, and the doctor ordered a Pap smear. Since they haven't seen an FGM female before, they were shocked to see what they found in me. I was ashamed of myself. I had to explain that it was done to me in my country. They asked if I had surgery. I told them it was part of my custom and tradition to initiate young girls into FGM to show that a young girl is matured and ready for womanhood. Several doctors came to see me and asked many questions. I was very uncomfortable, and because of that, I never want to go to another clinic.

Few weeks later, Felix took me to one of the vocational schools to see what courses I could enroll in. We agreed that I studied child-care. Since I enjoyed working with children, I enrolled for a childcare certificate program. It was a six-month program, and depending on your study habits and skills, it could be done sooner than six months. I finished it in no time! I got a job in a nursery school. I worked as a nursery school teacher and braided hair on my spare time.

In 1984, I became pregnant. We were both surprised as I was on the diaphragm birth control. Felix was extremely disappointed. He felt the pregnancy and baby would interfere with his studies and was not ready for the pregnancy. Because of his busy schedules he was not very supportive financially and emotionally during my pregnancy. In fact, he wanted me to have an abortion but I refused. To say the least, I had a very difficult time during my pregnancy. Felix refused to assist me most of the time and let me know that I wanted the pregnancy and I have to be responsible for it. I felt alone and had to take care of myself throughout. I missed home very much during this time as well because my families and friends would have supported me wholeheartedly during my pregnancy. Thankfully, some of my friends in Alumni Village including Julie helped me out a lot. Also, it was difficult to go to any doctor or a clinic as I was scared due to my previous experience with the medical folks trying to investigate my FGM. Anyhow, we found a lady who was a midwife, who worked at Planned Parenthood and she understood my plight. Apparently, she has worked with FGM women before. I was comfortable with her, and I continue to use her as my prenatal care person. On Monday, July 1, 1985, Leeann Mahota Rizk was born to Felix and me. This was one of the highest point in my marriage and my happiest. After my daughter's birth, our marriage problem took a deep! We encountered several turbulences. We persevered until Felix completed his master's degree and started his PhD in geology at FSU. I stayed home with Leeann and babysat other kids at home. Later, I worked for a very nice family in Tallahassee taking care of their two kids after school. They allowed me to bring Leeann along. In the morning, I attended a vocational school for an accounting clerical education course. Leeann was at the vocational school childcare and she was provided with childcare scholarship as well. I worked with this family for a couple of years.

Later that year, my younger sister, Comfort came to visit us from Sierra Leone. She stayed with us for a while. She decided to stay and live in the United States and didn't want to go back to Sierra Leone. Because Felix and I were constantly quarrelling, she was uncomfortable staying with us. She decided to move with some friends and relatives in Atlanta. Plus she enjoys bigger cities and thought Tallahassee was too small for her. I really didn't want her to go, but she didn't really like Tallahassee and the fact that Felix and I were always quarreling was not agreeable with her. Sadly, she moved away. It gave me an opportunity to visit Atlanta frequently. Since it is a bigger city than Tallahassee, there were more fun parties and gatherings there. We were invited and we went as much as we could.

Our marriage got really bad. So very difficult during these times in our marriage that we both decided that we send Leeann to Sierra Leone. When my eldest sister, Si Ebun, came to visit, we decided that she took Leeann with her to Sierra Leone. This way we can have time for school, work, and try to work our marital differences. When Si Ebun was leaving for Sierra Leone, Felix bought a ticket for Leeann to go with her. She was about a year and half. Foreign students will often send their children to their home countries while they pursue their education. So we thought we could do this as well.

I was depressed and cried about my decision! I knew we could manage with Leeann if we tried, but both Felix and I were stubborn and did not want to relent. When Leeann and my sister departed from Tallahassee, Si Ebun spent a few days in Atlanta and then a whole week in Washington DC. It was very difficult without Leeann that we both agreed to get Leeann back with us before my sister leaves the shore of America. Also, we had friends who were not really happy that we were sending our daughter away. They pressured us to bring her back and some were in favor as well. One particular friend, the late Alu (may his soul rest in peace) was against the idea of sending Leeann away. In fact, one day Alu and another friend had a serious bout of argument on the issue in our apartment. At the end of it, Felix and I decided to bring back Leeann. He got a one-day round-trip ticket for me to fly to Washington DC to go get Leeann and back. I got Leeann and flew back to Tallahassee in twenty-four hours. The return of Leeann brought some stability in our marriage and strengthened our relationship a bit. We regretted trying to send her off and we vouched never to do such in our marriage anymore. We agreed she is our responsibility and we should care for her. That was one great move we made in our relationship, and I am thankful up till today for that.

I continued with my business and accounting clerical skills training at Lively Technical College. I finished in one year and got a job with a state agency as an accounting clerk. Then I got pregnant again! This time, I asked Felix to agree that he will help me during the pregnancy and with the baby as well. I know he is busy with his PhD but I needed his assurance. He said that he doesn't have that time now and we should get an abortion. Reluctantly, I agreed and we aborted baby number three. Felix and I had the first abortion in Freetown, when he decided to test my eggs for fertility at the tender age of seventeen. He was in charge of making sure I did not get pregnant, naive me! I trusted him as an older guy and he was very controlling to say the least. However, he said he wanted to know that I could have babies so he did not protect our sexual activity. I got pregnant and it was very depressing for me! I had dreams of doing great things with education and I was disappointed at myself. Besides, this was only a year into our relationship. He was like twenty-nine years old and I was seventeen. But since he was a serious type of man who lectured at the college, my family thought he was good for me. I never showed or talked about his controlling side. Except, one time when he gave me a good beating and swear that I wanted him out of my life. But he engaged my friends and families. They pressured me into forgiving him. Those were big mistakes and I wish I had kept to my words and just left him. Anyhow, our first abortion took place.

For the third pregnancy, I had a friend that I confided with and she advised that I get the abortion as my husband was not a good husband. I trusted her judgment as she was married and it seems they had a good marriage. This is one of the biggest mistakes of my life that I regret up to today. Because I should have sacrificed and kept the baby! I learned later from most married couples that the wives or mothers are the foundation in the children's life. Most times fathers are busy with their stuff and mothers are with the children. I mean, I saw that in my mother's days but I didn't want that for me. That was a great reality check for me! Because up to today, I see the same trends as mothers are always the children's keepers! Nowadays, when I see young people who go through teenage pregnancy and survived as well as achieving success, I feel very guilty of having abortions. Even though I was a teenager, I would have made it. Oh well, it is what it is! I didn't tell my good friend, Julie, about the second pregnancy at the time as I knew she would have convinced me not to go through with the abortion. Later, when I confided in her and told her of the pregnancy, she was mad with me and she said that she would have convinced me to keep it. During her marriage to her husband, she had her second child even though her marriage was on the edge. Today, she has two beautiful and helpful girls with several grandchildren. If I had kept those pregnancies, I would have three children today. I am often sad about it as my dreams were to have a few babies. Since this time, I vouched to always convince women to abstain from abortions. I feel it is a heavy lifelong guilt and one feels as if one killed his or her child. Additionally, childbearing is a gift from God, and I believe that he makes a way for everyone to raise their children when they try.

Around that same time, Julie had got a job and she relocated to Albany, New York. She was concerned about my well-being and we agreed that I moved with her to Albany to see if I could be happier and comfortable living there. I quit my job in Florida and moved to Albany. I got a job right away at Walmart. Julie would drop me off to work and pick me up. She and the girls will babysit Leeann for me as well. It was working well. I dated an Italian guy who really liked me. He would take me to work and back. Our relationship was very platonic! Julie's mother stepped in as a mother and grandmother as well. She would give me valuable advises especially when Julie was not around. May her gentle soul rest in perfect peace! One day she visited Leeann and I in the morning when everyone had gone to work and/ or school and talked me into returning back to my husband and save our marriage! Additionally, Leeann missed her daddy too.

After about three months away, we moved back to Tallahassee. Our relationship got worse. I caught him cheating with one of his female students and we had many bouts hence forth. After many of these bouts, I lost a lot of weight and almost drove myself insane. I remembered chasing Felix and the girlfriend with a machete. Felix and the girlfriend called the police and I was arrested. Tormented and confused, I didn't know where to turn. I burst out weeping in the police car. All of a sudden the police pulled over and talked to me. He said that he knew I was desperate but I couldn't take the law into my hands. He said it doesn't work that way in America and that I could be jailed for a very a long time. We made a deal that I must leave Tallahassee and that was the only way he would let me go. He gave me twenty-four hours to leave the city of Tallahassee. I gave him my sister, Comfort's phone number and he called her and explained the situation. Comfort drove to Tallahassee the next morning. We packed my stuff and left town. Felix filed for a divorce. Leeann and I lived in Atlanta for over a year. I was twenty-seven years old then. I moved on and even dated a few people. I was really ready to move on. There was a gentle man I met who really was ready to marry me right away. After our divorce, Felix was sure that he was going to marry the German student he was dating. I was not hopeful for reconciliation at all. Again, Leeann missed her dad and pleaded that we go back to Tallahassee. Felix missed us too and pleaded that we returned home. After a series of negotiations which included that he abandoned his relationship with the student, we agreed to go back to Tallahassee. We decided to have another wedding and start afresh all over again. So we had the wedding and invited our friends and relatives. I prayed that our marriage turbulences were over and we could live in peace.

This is now 1991 and he graduated with a PhD in Geology and Oceanography. Also, he was working for a formidable geology company in Tallahassee. However his dream job was to become a professor in Geology. Luckily, he got a job in Iowa and we moved to Cedar Falls, Iowa. My niece, Fatu Forna, had just come to live with us during this time. All four of us—Felix, Fatu, Leeann, and I made the move and long drive to Iowa. To be honest, I didn't want or like the move. To make him happy and because he was the breadwinner, I went with the flow and so are the kids. But living in Cedar Falls was a bit hellish. We were lonely. So we spent a lot of time at the local YMCA. Fatu and Leeann took up swimming and I worked out on the equipment. I even got a trainer! However, our relationship continued to be in turmoil. I was able to adjust to Iowa and found a job in a day care center as the secretary and child caregiver. I enjoyed it and the kids and I were adjusting okay. We dreaded the cold harsh winter months and we were not looking forward to it. Really didn't want to leave Tallahassee but Felix was the main provider so we go wherever he goes. After about a year in Iowa, Felix had many fracases with the university he worked for and he said he doesn't want to work with them anymore. Iowa was not ready for an African American professor and they were very prejudice. Felix didn't handle it well and we had to leave. Thankfully, his job in Tallahassee hired him right back. He was smart and always an asset in his professions. I stayed in Cedar Falls so my niece and daughter could finish the school year. Fatu was in twelfth grade and she was doing exceptionally well. She got admission into Florida Agriculture and Marine University (FAMU). Leeann had a rough school year as the kids were shocked to have a colored girl in their class. Some treated her well and others not so good. She survived and was promoted to first grade. All of us were excited to move back to Tallahassee after our bittersweet experience with the weather and Iowa as a whole.

As soon as I got back to Tallahassee, I began job hunting and trying to head back to college to work on my degree. My sister, Comfort, got very ill during her second pregnancy where she suffered a stroke. Since I was not working and I was job searching, Felix and I agreed that I could move to Atlanta for a few a months to assist her. So I left Leeann with Felix and went to Atlanta. The good thing is that Comfort had a childcare job that I was able to work and earn money. Felix or me will visit once or two times a month during my absent. Our relationship was really rocky too but I wanted to assist my sister as well. Apparently, while I was in Iowa, Felix dated a woman from his work and they were getting serious as he told her he wasn't married. Also, we bought our first home at the same time. I insisted to Felix that I wanted to see the house papers as I was away when he purchased the house. When I saw the papers of the house, it stated Felix was not married and no kids. I was very upset and confronted him. He didn't have much to say about it. He said that he did that because it was easier and faster to buy the house this way. I was very upset. I never wanted to stay in that house anymore. I felt violated! Especially when I placed my personal funds that I saved up into buying the house for us! Anyway, I worked Comfort's job and made some money while assisting her to get through her illness in Atlanta. I cheated and dated an old boyfriend who later became my second husband. Upon my return to Tallahassee, our relationship went so bad that I moved out and got my own apartment for the first time. One of the last straws that break the camel's back for me in our marriage was when, we were trying to have another baby and I couldn't get pregnant. Then Felix said to me that if I don't fix whatever problem I have, he will leave me and find another woman who could have him some babies. I thought he was serious about it as he lost interest in the relationship completely and was not trying to improve. I was tired and I was trying to find a way out. I enrolled at Tallahassee Community College to work on an associate's degree in General Studies. We tried counseling but nothing worked. My husband was cheating. We had immigration problems as we did not have residency in the United States. Felix thought the only way to have his immigration rectified was to divorce me and marry an American who will make his papers legal. So he filed for divorce and went on to pursue his dreams with another woman.

I continued with my studies at Tallahassee Community College. This time, instead of running away from Tallahassee, I stayed and faced all my problems. I got an apartment and got my American residency rectified. I got a job with the Florida State Department of Education, where I worked for more than ten years and was vested into the Florida Retirement System. It was hard, so I took another break. This time I decided to study something for fun. So I took courses in cosmetology, nail technology and took classes on makeup and facial care. I always wanted to do these courses but my ex-husband did not approve of me doing them so I could not pursue it. After our separation and final divorce, I pursued the courses and received my certificates in a year. That year, I celebrated my thirtieth birthday as well. That same year, I made my first visit to Sierra Leone for the first time after twelve years.

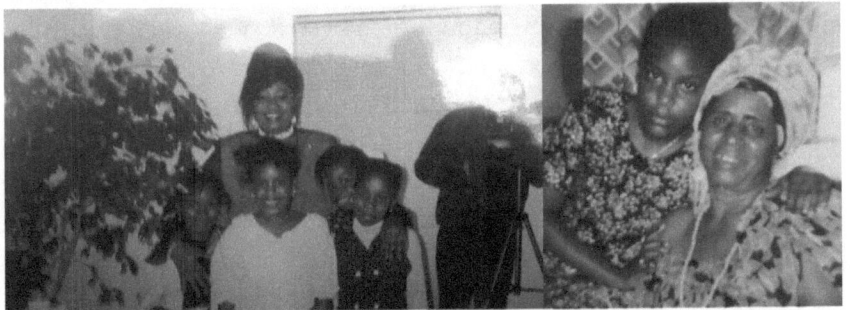

Lola's thirtieth birthday picture   Leeann and Mama
1994 Freetown

Sierra Leone was fun and it was nice to see my families, friends, and everyone. I was able to connect with some folks that I needed to make amends with. They were all happy to see me. The best thing from my visit was that I was able to get a visiting visa for my mother to visit the United States. I returned back to the United States with our mom in January 1995 and it was just amazing traveling with her on that very long journey. We flew from Sierra Leone to Europe and we landed in Atlanta, Georgia. She was hilarious during the trip and made us laugh throughout the journey. One incidence that I still laugh about was her first experience with the escalator! She thought it was easy and much like a staircase. Mind you, our mom suffers from polio so she generally needs helps to get along. Really wished she used a cane but never did for fear of the stigmatization or labeling that goes with carrying a stick, so she went on without using canes. She tried to get on the escalators and she quickly called for help and grabbed me as her feet were spreading apart faster than she could handle. It was very funny because I had a similar experience traveling to America for the first time. Only that I was alone and strangers came to my rescue. Upon our arrival in the States, mom stayed with Comfort in Atlanta for a while then I picked her up later.

We arrived in the USA in January 1995. After that year, the Sierra Leone Civil War went ballistic. That war lasted for more than ten years. It was a good thing that our mother was out of the country during the war. Many people were left amputated and they lost their limbs and or arms. Houses were burnt down and looted. My childhood home was burnt down and looted as well. We lost all our childhood pictures and treasures; hence I have none of them to share. My family in Sierra Leone suffered great atrocities. Young females were raped and kidnapped. One of my nieces was kidnapped and taken to the war zone by the rebels. They kidnapped many young girls and boys. The girls became sexual mates while the young boys were used as soldiers. The war resulted to the birth of many child soldiers. Sierra Leone was a war-torn nation for a while and it took the country backward in decades. The country suffered major brain drain as many professionals and educated people flee the country seeking greener pastures in other parts of the world. In the early 2000s, it got better. People started to return home slowly and visitors came back slowly to Sierra Leone as well.

Upon completion of the cosmetology and nail programs, I decided to go back to the community college to finish up my associate degree. I graduated from Tallahassee Community College in 1996 and mom was there to witness that beautiful event. That very same year I bought and owned my first house. Meanwhile, Felix and I were separated. In 1997 I filed for a divorce and moved on with my life. By this time, I have a childcare certificate, business and accounting certificate, cosmetology, beauty and nail technology certificates, and an associate degree from Tallahassee Community College. During this time, I negotiated with my daughter that she go and live with my sister and my mom in Atlanta for little a while until I could sort out some issues in my life and finish with the cosmetology. We agreed but at the end of it Leeann was very unhappy. That was one move I regretted! My daughter did not like it and I did not like it either. Up till now, we still talk about it, and she despised that experience. I pleaded with her and asked her to forgive me for doing that. At that time, I was going through some difficult times in my life, and I needed that time to sort my life. Luckily, my mom was around, and I trusted her to keep a close eye on her at my sister's. Additionally, she and my sister's kids are much like siblings and they get along very well. In fact every summer, they would spend it with us in Florida. So I thought she would be okay. She was, but she missed her mother, and we know there is no one like a Mom! Also, she and my sister were cool, but my sister is very strong headed, and they butt heads during those times as well. They are really cool with each other. In fact, she often tells me that she feels very close to that my sister and family than any of my other siblings. Even though I made sure we saw each other at least once a month by using Air South, which was a shuttle between Atlanta and Tallahassee and very affordable at the time. Sometimes a ticket would cost $29 one way! So I would buy tickets for all the kids, and my mother to come for a long weekend or a break. It worked out well. Other times I would drive to Atlanta, which was only four hours away from Tallahassee. Leeann said that she was unhappy without me in Atlanta. So I tried my best and brought her back to Tallahassee in less than a year later. She despises that separation up till today. It brought memories of when we wanted to send her to Sierra Leone and we got her from my sister at the airport in Washington DC. I had vouched not to separate from her but I had to. We continue to weather the storm with it!

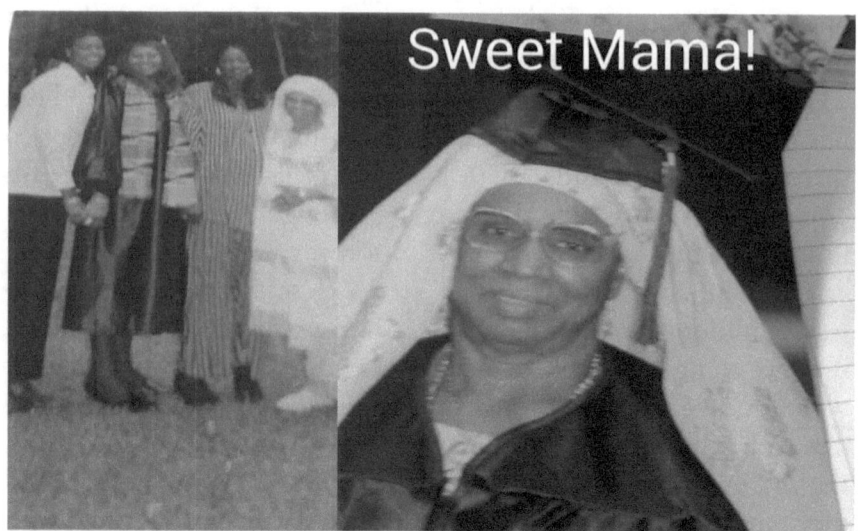

Leeann, Me, Hoaua, and Mom: Mom with my graduation
cap and gown. "She graduated too," she says.

2

Diagnosis and Reactions

Acquiring all these educations and dealing with the traumas of early marriage, sexual, emotional and physical child abuses along with the impacts of FGM may have taken a toll in my life. It seems like I am always trying to prove a point to the world and those who left me broken! I worked very hard as well as very long hours trying to prove myself and I started to get tired and exhausted. I began to feel sick all the time! Doctors couldn't pinpoint my diagnosis. I feel tired all the time, helpless. I lost lots of weight and I lost hair. I looked frail! Sometimes, I would just collapse and just pass out for no reason. For instance, I will feel dizzy, and before I know it, I am in an ambulance or people are trying to help me out. It was embarrassing at times! I never understood why and I was very worried about myself at one point that I went through a depression stage. I had to be medicated for depression at some point. But the medications made me feel suicidal so I stopped taking them. I had to do several blood tests and health checkups. Thankfully, I had a state job with very good health benefits that was a savior. I remembered having to do a liver biopsy as well. All the results were promising except for some lipids in my liver. I ended up taking steroids like prednisone, Plaquenil, and other immunosuppressant. I have been taking them ever since. There was a lady who was my first lupus known case, I called her Mother Teresa. She told me she had signs similar to mine and she was taking similar drugs like I was taking. She helped me during my liver biopsy, took me into her home, and cared for me during and after my surgery. Mrs. Janice Leland, may her gentle soul continue to rest in perfect peace. She was the first one to enlighten me about lupus. After her death, I thought quietly to myself that lupus will get me next, but I prayed as well as did what the doctors ordered. Thankfully, I am still here! No family member of mine had it. Except my dad, who showed signs of it as I recalled. But lupus is so hard to understand as a disease everywhere and even in the United States at that time. So it is hard to diagnose it, and it's even more difficult to diagnose in Africa given its limited health opportunities.

My mother came to live with me to help me out during these difficult times. However, I continue to get sicker. She helped out a lot! My cousin-in-law Haoua Barrie also lived with me along with one of my younger half-sisters, Joko, and her five-year-old daughter Tina. I always had family members around. My house was always open to families and friends as well as very welcoming. During this time, I was a student at Florida State University completing my degree in business with a major in marketing and minor in French.

In early 1998, I was finally diagnosed with lupus. It was a shocker! I was devastated, and I was in denial. Around this time, Mom was leaving as she was getting ready to return to Sierra Leone as the war ended. She missed her families and friends very much. It was only fair that she goes. My cousin-in-law and her newborn baby, Mica, were leaving as well to join her husband in Virginia Beach. Also, my half-sister and her daughter had moved out as well. With this new diagnosis, I was afraid to live with just my daughter and me. It was rough! Leeann and I managed our lives in Tallahassee. In early 1999, I was able to get six months of sick leave from the state government that I worked for. Later that year, I got a scholarship to do a three months' study abroad program in France. I met a great colleague and friend on my Paris trip. Her name is Rawan! It has been a pleasure to know her and up till now we are still buddies. I left Tallahassee in June and return in August. Leeann was able to spend a whole month in Europe with me. She met me in Paris, and we went to Disneyland Paris together as well as London. We had a great and memorable summer.

We returned back in August to get Leeann back to school and I was getting ready for college as well. Leeann and I discussed that I will need to be near family due to my illness and we agreed to move to Atlanta. Leeann finished up tenth grade at Chiles High School in Tallahassee. She finished in summer of 2001. In order for her not to miss out on the school year we agreed that she would spend a semester without me in Atlanta. This time, she lived with Fatu, my doctor niece, and two of my oldest nieces; they were both in high school. So it wasn't so bad, and she was older as well. Plus, I was coming back by the end of the semester. We spent most of the summer together though. I enrolled her in her new school. This time around she had a great time and did not regret at all. Leeann moved to Atlanta to start eleventh grade in Georgia. In December 2001, upon my graduation from Florida State University, I moved to Atlanta too. In Atlanta, I got a job with Emory University and worked there for about three years.

My daughter graduated from high school in May 2003. She got accepted to Florida Agriculture and Marine University (FAMU) where she pursued a degree in health-care management. For her graduation from high school, I gifted her with a brand-new vehicle. She drove it in Atlanta for about six months. Then in September 2003, I drove her in her car to Tallahassee and dropped her off at college. We decorated her room and I left her in the hands of God. It was very sad and difficult departing time but we did it. She was born in Tallahassee and it is a familiar place for her, so I thought she could be safe. Indeed, she was as she had many good supports. She found her way easily and she survived. She graduated four years later. Her graduation day was a momentous day for me. I was full of pride, joy, and happiness, to see my baby graduating along with some of her friends. I threw her a very big party and invited friends from all over the world. My families and friends came to support us big time!

While Leeann was a student in Tallahassee and I was living in Atlanta, I dated and married my second husband in 2003. He was someone that I previously dated. But broke up with him due to his womanizing and smoking habits. But we rekindled our relationship a second time around. I was particularly impressed that he went cold turkey on cigarettes! This time around he seemed more serious and I thought that he may have changed for the better even with womanizing. I was not really looking or trying to be in a serious relationship while I was raising Leeann and trying to send her off to college. As I really didn't want to move her anywhere else except for college and so I did. Upon my marriage, I moved to Maryland in June 2003, while Leeann was in Florida finishing up with college. We managed to see each other at least one or two times a year until she graduated in 2007.

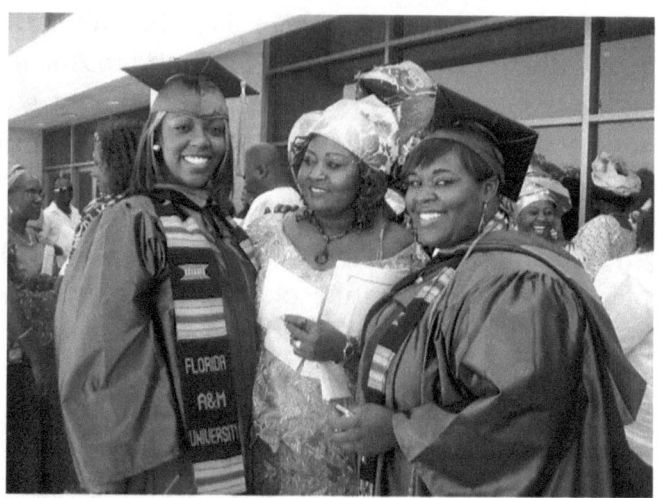

Leeann, me, and Kera (college BFF) Leeann, Uncle Martin, and me Leeann's graduation and party pictures L

3

Battles

Battle No. 1

In Maryland, I was married and lived with my second husband. I got a job at Georgetown University. During my stay in Maryland, I had a turbulent marriage again. Mainly because my husband continued with his infidelity activities and he has several baby mamas. The exes were constantly harassing me and my husband. All of a sudden, he stayed in the streets and hardly ever home. It was rough and I was much stressed. The fact that I had less family and friend support in Maryland made it even harder! The situation was very difficult on my lupus. I had and experienced my very first major battle with lupus during this period. I started to get sicker again dealing with the stress in my marriage and the new environment in Maryland. The good thing is that I found very good doctors at Kaiser Permanente in Maryland and they were very good and thorough in assisting me with my battle with lupus. For the first time I had a lung biopsy too. They found that I had interstitial lung disease and I needed to be on steroids. So they increased my prednisone. The doctor said that the prednisone will slow down my lung disease which is like scarring of the lung tissues. So I continued with prednisone, Plaquenil and Prilosec. I need these medications to manage my lupus and the lung disease. In addition, I was prescribed two liters of oxygen added to my medical treatment as well. My doctors advised that I need to find ways to eliminate stress in my life. It was difficult to do. The husband I moved there for was very uncooperative!

One time I was ill that 911 had to be called to pick me up. I was on the phone with one of my good friends, Isata Jalloh, and all of a sudden I blacked out. For the life of me, I don't know the rest of the story and I found myself in an ambulance. While on the phone with my friend, she realized I had problems as she is a nurse. She lived in New Jersey at the time. She called 911 from New Jersey and they break into my apartment to get me out. I didn't even know that one could call 911 from out of state to save a life! It was a blessing to speak with her at the time. That husband of mine could not be located until days after. I mean he stayed out all the time! Luckily, my sister, Ade, lived in New York City so she came to see me and spent time with me as much as she could. My husband at the time was very absent and was hardly ever around.

Later in April 2007, my daughter graduated from FAMU with a degree in Health Care Management. Soon after, she got a job in New York City. She moved to New York and lived with my sister. This move brought her very close to Maryland so we saw each other quite often. She would visit and I would visit her more in New York. Those were good times and I handled my lupus even better. I spent my birthdays and most holidays in New York City as it was my happy and less-stress zone. So I come to visit as often as I could. My husband visited once or twice with me but after that, he was always missing in action. I got used to his absence and lived as though I wasn't married.

I found out that Georgetown would give me fee waiver to do my masters at the university. While I was going through these trials, I was working on my masters at Georgetown. It was not easy. My long-time friend, Julie Goodwin, from Tallahassee had a job in education in Albany, New York. We got to see each other more often and she played a pertinent role in assisting me with my master's degree and writing my thesis. My thesis was focused on helping Sierra Leone in development. It was a good foundation to my future endeavors in Sierra Leone. So I did a case study on youth development in Sierra Leone. My friend, Dr. Julie Godwin, played a key role in helping me to accomplish this task. I made several trips to Albany and she came down to Maryland several times as well. We both worked hard on my thesis. I started working on my master's in January 2006 and graduated in May 2008 with a master's in International Studies from Georgetown University.

During my hospitalization period, I would work on finishing up my master's thesis. So at the hospital, I spent most of the time writing and finishing up on my sick bed. I wrote and e-mailed drafts of my thesis to my professors and Dr. Goodwin at the same time. It was rough but I pulled it through. The graduation was awesome. My sisters, Ade and Comfort, came including Haoua, Mika, and Fatima Barrie, Isata Jalloh, Dr. Julia Goodwin (friends), and my daughter Leeann Rizk. It was a beautiful day!

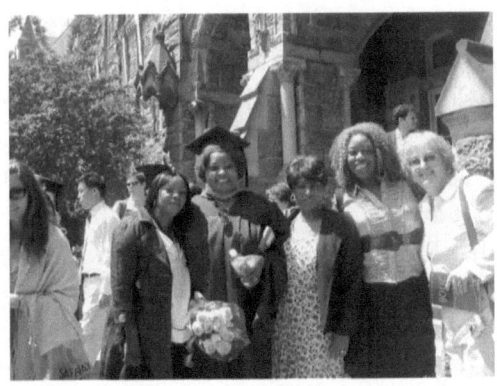

My daughter continued to stay with my older sister, Mrs. Ade Lekoetje, in New York City. She works for the United Nations. She was a great asset to us and helped both Leeann and I immensely. My trips to the Big Apple were many because of them. After a year, my marriage went from bad to worse. My husband had numerous affairs. He fathered a child while we were married and he already had about six other children with different women. He actually gave me a sexually transmitted disease and I thought, *Enough is enough, this relationship was over!* I was faced with another divorce. I continue to have challenges with lupus and the interstitial lung disease. However, I had great doctors and I was assured to get better. After working for Georgetown for five years, I decided to pack up and leave. I moved out of his house and lived with my cousin in Maryland. Then I filed for a divorce from him. In about a year, the divorce became final. I was feeling better and really enjoying life. I joined the YMCA gym and I exercised faithfully. I felt like lupus was gone for good! So I decided to move back to my family in Atlanta. While in Atlanta, I made up my mind to move back to Sierra Leone to render my expertise and services in education, which was highly needed in the country. Since my lupus was kind of dormant at the time and I off-loaded the bad marriage and its stresses, I felt that it was a good time to make my move to Sierra Leone. Also, I wanted to give back my services to my mother's land, as well as spend some time with my mom too.

I still have my house in Florida then, and my brother and his family lived in it. It was a battle to get them out of the house. Long story but it was eventually done and the house was sold. The money from that sale and the money I received from Georgetown and Emory Universities, the government of Florida, and any other benefits I collected assisted me with my move to Sierra Leone. Luckily for me, lupus was away and I was feeling my best ever. I continue to have a feeling that lupus was gone for good! I really wanted to return home and the feeling of returning home got even bigger for me. At age forty-two, I moved to Sierra Leone. I was very excited about my decision. My daughter was worried about me, but she wanted me to be happy. She decided to take a week off to fly with me to Sierra Leone and help me settle down. It was nice to have her with me as I try to make the move. Leeann was worried about me settling and she thought she could help. She was a huge help. Also, many of my relatives were very supportive in helping with my move. My mother was exceptionally happy and I was happy to spend some time with her. My sisters, cousins, aunties, uncles, nieces, and nephews were exceptional. Mam, my little niece, who stayed with us was very gracious and very helpful. Really, my families were awesome. Sierra Leone was a great move for me, and I treasured it. As soon as Leeann felt I was comfortable, she left after a few weeks to return to work in New York City.

Six months later, my daughter decided to move to Sierra Leone to explore work opportunities. She was interested in the Peace Corps program, but it didn't happen, so she wanted to do some service work in Sierra Leone. She volunteered at Marie Stopes, a health-care nongovernmental organization. She volunteered for about six months and she was given a paid job at Marie Stopes as Health Care Coordinator. She enjoyed it and it was much like a Peace Corp type opportunity program. She travelled all over the country too.

I managed lupus very well in Sierra Leone. Si Ebun, the eldest sister in the family provided a home for us in Sierra Leone. We stayed in Sierra Leone for a whole year before we came to visit America in June 2009. We had a great time. I did a complete medical physical examination while we were visiting the United States, I made sure that I got all my medications and had a checkup. My daughter got ill on this visit. We thought she had malaria. A doctor friend of mine advised that we do a pregnancy test before treating for anything. We did the test, and indeed, she was pregnant! Although, she had a boyfriend in Sierra Leone but because she was not married, she was concerned and worried. I was a bit disappointed too as I wanted her to be married before having a child. We spoke to the boyfriend and informed him about the pregnancy. He told us that he would support any decision we take in regard to the pregnancy. I convinced Leeann to keep the pregnancy and she did. We enjoyed the rest of our holidays and returned back to Sierra Leone.

At this time, I worked at the University of Sierra Leone (USL) as the planning director. Later I worked as the head of public relations for the USL. I also wrote several grants and launched several programs in youth development. I introduced professional seminars to develop student professionalism and get them ready for a career. Students were coached on resume writing, taught them basic office business skills, writing memorandum, interviewing skills, and many other professional best practices. Additionally, I introduced the job fair scheme for college graduates. I also ran programs for high schools to get them acquainted with college requirements and to prepare them for college. With the help of a very prominent lady, Mrs. Kona Koroma, who is for education and development in Sierra Leone, we were able to sell such program to the government of Sierra Leone, United Nations Development Programme (UNDP) of Sierra Leone

and the Sierra Leone National Youth Commission (NAYCOM).
These organizations partnered with the USL and we established
a center that was named the USL Career Advising and Placement
Services (CAPS). It empowered many graduates. Due to the need
for such programs in the country, the NAYCOM, UNDP, and the
Ministry of Education created a national internship program, where
I played a key role in ensuring youths in Sierra Leone were empowered. Up to today, I still have relationships with students in Sierra
Leone. I have helped them grow professionally and they are all over
the world. Sometimes they send their resumes and documents via
e-mail to me to edit for them up till now. I do so happily and no
charge.

Additionally, I had the opportunity to meet with great per-
sonalities like the president of my country His Excellency President
Earnest Bai Koroma, Prime Minister Tony Blair, and many other
diplomats in the Sierra Leone community including ambassadors of
many countries. I assisted in launching several programs at the USL.
One big program we launched was the Confucius College at Fourah
Bay College. This program introduced Sierra Leoneans to Chinese
cultures in Sierra Leone. Students were taken to China on exchange
programs as well. Chinese language was taught in Sierra Leone as
well.

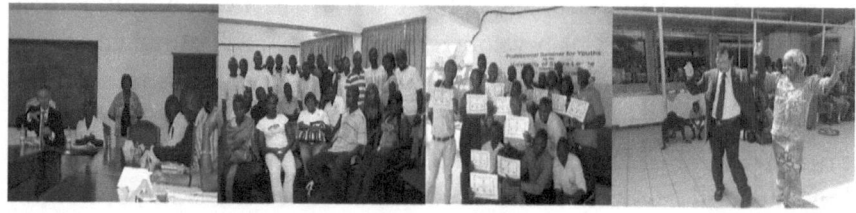

A picture with His Excellency Mr. Tony Blair and a cross section
of students who benefited from the professional programs organized
at USL and a dance to celebrate Confucius College launch

In February 2010, my daughter came to USA to give birth. I
joined her later to support her through the process. Chernor Malik
Bah, the joy of my life was born on April 8, 2010. We stayed in the

United States just enough time for him to get all his first checkups and we got our tickets, packed our bags, and came back to Sierra Leone. I made sure that I did all my health checks as well as took care of my medications. I returned back to Sierra Leone in good health.

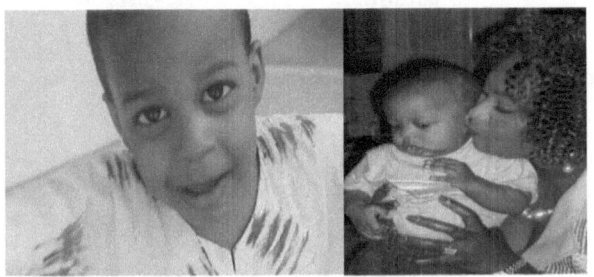

Photos of Malik and me

Battle No. 2

Although I was battling lupus well, the pollution and lack of good medical conditions did not sit well with lupus in Sierra Leone. In early 2011, I got sick and had to rush to the United States for treatment. I was feeling real bad and lupus seem to be active again. I flew from Freetown to Atlanta. Upon my arrival in Atlanta Airport, Comfort picked me. I was feeling very bad, and I asked her to please take me to the ER at Grady Memorial Hospital. I was admitted for one week. It was rough and my hospital stay seemed endless. There were signs of progression of my lung disease and flair of lupus. I was given medications and I was discharged. They also prescribed inhalers as well. Thank God I came! After about three weeks in Atlanta, I felt better and returned back to Sierra Leone. As soon as I arrived, the seminars and other programs had to be done, so I jumped on it and it was done. I felt rejuvenated and well. Although some of my good friends advised me to think about returning back to the United States, I was enjoying Sierra Leone and wanted to see how far I could stretch it. Anyway, I went to Sierra Leone and did all my work as planned. We celebrated Malik's first birthday in April 2011.

My daughter and her husband left Sierra Leone in October 2011 to relocate to New York City. Malik was left with me in Freetown. The plan was that Malik would join them later when they are settled with work and got an apartment. They stayed with a good friend and sister of my daughter, Mrs. Pauline Pratt, who was very helpful to them as they were trying to establish in New York City.

Battle No. 3

By the end of 2011, I got very ill again in Sierra Leone. I managed lupus in Sierra Leone but the doctors do not really know how to treat it and they are not sure of the right medications. Honestly, even in the United States it was a difficult task for the doctors. I often feel like it's a trial-and-error-based treatment. Finally, I flew out of Sierra Leone for the USA again in February 2012 and brought along my grandson. We arrived safely and Comfort picked us up from Atlanta Airport. She drove me to Gwinnett County Hospital Emergency Room right away as my health was very shaky and she wasn't comfortable taking me home. I was admitted right away and I stayed in the hospital there for a week. I had brought my grandson with me because his parents were not in Sierra Leone and I was not comfortable leaving him behind. We stayed in Georgia with Comfort for about three months. Later we came to New York City to join Malik's parents as they settled down and have their own apartment.

During my hospitalization at Gwinnett Hospital, the hospital advised that I consider filing for Medicaid and Medicare as lupus is a chronic and life-threatening illness. They said that I will need constant health care. I did not take the advice seriously as I wanted to go back to Sierra Leone. I was working on several projects in Sierra Leone and they needed to be done. I was running CAPS for college graduates of the USL and it was time to have the workshops. It is usually a two-phase event. The professional seminars, where we coach students on resume writing and getting them ready for the professional world. We use newspapers to look at newspaper job advertisements and how to respond to them by doing letters. We also look at thank you letters along with application letters as well as dressing for success in a professional manner and other professional best practices. All participants were given a certificate at the end of the seminar.

At the job fair, business organizations of all types—governmental, nongovernmental, banks, and private industries were present and it was quite successful. It is sort of a business trade fair for business. It provided an opportunity for young people to learn about the business in Sierra Leone and how to network with them for professional opportunities. The good thing is that the students were all professionally ready as they were groomed through the professional seminar. I was also working on a national internship program with the NAYCOM, the Minister of Education, and UNDP that was been launched. So my returning home to assist with these projects was eminent. It all went well and I delivered successfully. I was happy, relaxed, and thankful. In addition to these events, I partnered with Bolo Spencer Coker to do entrepreneurship workshops for the graduates as well. It was very successful and wetted the appetites of young people to become entrepreneurs. Today, some of these students run their own businesses and others are doing well professionally.

So I jumped on an airplane as soon as I felt better again and off to Sierra Leone I go! Malik stayed in New York City with his parents. Before leaving, I helped secure a very nice childcare for him. I also helped him make the transition. It was difficult for him. But he got use to his new set up and that made me happy. It was difficult to leave without Malik for me as well. But I had no choice as SiEbun, whose house we lived in didn't think I should bring back Malik because of my health situation. Also, she feels like Malik should be with his parents. However, Pateh and Leeann were not quite ready for Malik as they were still adjusting to living in New York. They had no choice but to make the accommodations to keep their child as I couldn't take him back with me even if I wanted to. I helped them a lot in the past and I feel they would manage henceforth. In any case, it is their child and I needed to live my life too. Both Pateh and Leeann were raised well and now they have the chance to raise their own. They are doing a fine job so far so good!

People who suffer from lupus usually have rheumatoid arthritis issues. My right arm, which I use for everything, had rheumatoid issues. It hurts a lot and it was swelling. At night I couldn't sleep as it burns and constantly aches. I drank Ibuprofen for the pain all the time and sometimes I place a band over it. I need that hand for writing; typing and you name it, so I didn't want it to go bad on me. It was my stronger hand as a right-handed person. My third sibling—Feyi, who has lived in Sierra Leone for most of her life—understands the system in Sierra Leone better than most people in my family. She is my go-to person for many things. Even as a young person, I thought she was street-smarter than most people in my family. In fact, when I had my first pregnancy and abortion experience as a young girl, she was the only family member I confided in. She and Felix were the only two people present by my side. So when I got to Freetown, she was more of my confidant! But nowadays, we are at loggerheads for whatever reasons, I am not sure of. I keep our relationship in prayers and often ask our angel mother to intercede. Anyway, Feyi recommended a doctor to look at my arm. The same doctor had done surgery on her once. Since I trusted her judgment and recommendation, I decided to try her doctor. So I saw the doctor and he looked at my arm and said it was a ganglion cyst! Although in the United States I was told it was rheumatoid nodules! The doctor in Sierra Leone said he could operate on it. Without X-ray or MRI, he looked at it and set up the surgery. I was happy as I thought that my pains and swelling would go away and he promised me that too. Since I have lung issues, I was told in the United States to avoid general anesthesia. So I told the doctor to use only anesthetic to the arm and mild sedation to get me relaxed. That's what they did and we headed for the operating theater.

During surgery I could hear the discussions but couldn't speak. I heard the doctor said, "Oh no, it's not." after he cut me opened. I could feel the cutting like cutting of my nerve but it wasn't painful. So he said they would leave it alone. It was a painful recovery. I went to see him for my follow-up and he told me that it wasn't what he thought and it seems it's something else. So he was unable to remove it completely. So he got some tissues that need to be examined. We had to send it to South Africa through a testing laboratory and I had to pay for the cost of that. In a week, the result came back to say it is rheumatoid nodules that may have come from my lupus. I was left with a huge scar that is still visible. Since that day, I decided no serious surgery or medical stuff for me and lupus in Sierra Leone except if I want to die soonest! Plus my daughter was very angry that I took such a chance given my health situation.

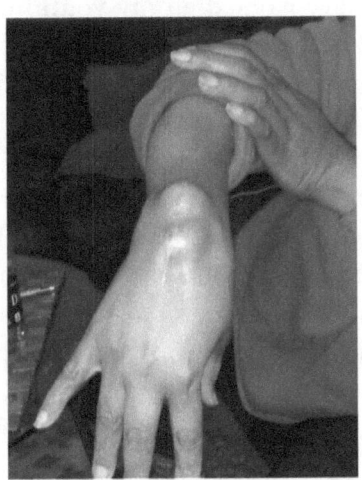

My arm with rheumatoid nodules

Battle No. 4

Sadly, as soon as I finished with all the projects and feeling better with the hand, I began to feel sick again. I packed my suitcases and off to Atlanta as all my medical records were kept there. My colleague and friend, Dr. Lauretta Sillah, and her daughter Yasa picked me up at the Atlanta Airport. From the airport we went directly to Grady Hospital. I was so sick that I was placed in the intensive care unit. I was in a lot of pain and couldn't breathe. I was placed on an oxygen machine to help me with my breathing. This time, I stayed in the United States for about six months. I finally decided to file for medical help and it was offered to me. With a chronic illness like lupus, I need health insurance all the time. I got better and came to New York City and visited with my daughter and family. For the first time I started to rethink my idea about my decision to move back to Sierra Leone and that it might not work for lupus and me! I may need to consider moving back to the USA and/or visit more often or do consultancies. I was a bit depressed over this and worried. I handed it over to God almighty as the driver of my life and pray that he orders my steps in his words. Really, America has good medical facilities and I have worked all my youthful days in the USA. I have invested in the health and retirement system that I haven't done in Sierra Leone. Moreover, I am comfortable living in the United States but home is home and I wanted to go back. Soon, I realize that home is really where one is most comfortable and so the move back to the States may have to be! Soon after I felt better, I came to New York and visited with Leeann and family. I played with Malik a bit and even visited his school and read stories about Sierra Leone to the kids. I am very good with kids as I took a childcare course in Florida to work as a child caregiver. I visited his preschool and Malik was thrilled. Had a quick but quality visit with them and off I go to Sweet Sierra Leone!

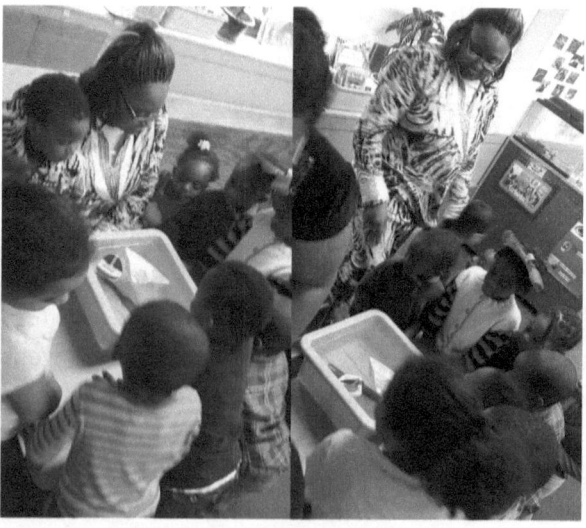

Volunteering at Malik's School

I returned back to Sierra Leone as I had many unfinished business to take care of. One such business was the Miss University of Sierra Leone Beauty Pageant. I participated as one of the coordinators representing the universities. Africa Young Voices (AYV) organization was the organizer of the pageants and I worked with them. They had sent a letter requesting that I participate in the university pageant and it was approved by the USL head. That year's pageant was hectic as it had many conflicts. One of the mothers of the contestants was against her participation in the competition. She believed that a beauty pageant was a way to expose young girls to prostitution and negative behaviors. She tried to drag the pageant's platform down the drain via the media. She specifically mentioned my name in the conversations on the media. Because I had empathy for the girl who wants to experience pageantry, I decided to take her under my wings and helped her as much as I could. The CEO of AYV and I had to defend the pageant on the air as well. The head of the USL at that time was negative about the university pageant as well and was against student participation. However, the university pageant is meant for college and university students. Girl students who are doing well academically and are over the age of eighteen are welcome to submit an application of participation. But the head of the USL thought that pageants were distractions and only girls who are not serious participate in pageants. We had an argument over it and I tried to defend the pageants but it did not sit well with him. Anyway, that year's pageant had the most fracases! In retrospect, the mother may have known her daughter very well as her daughter proved to be a slut! For the most part, most of the participants were sober, hardworking, and participated in good faith with intentions to win and explore other opportunities.

Right after the university pageants is usually the All Walks of Life (AWOL) award program. This award takes a deeper look at different organizations and how well they serve the people and they are awarded for exceling in the country. I was on the board to represent the educational facilities and to coordinate between the universities and AWOL. It's usually a huge celebration. Every business is looked at and ranked as well as voted for by the people of Sierra Leone. It ends with a grand finale as well. It is a lot of work! Both of the projects are under AYV. I was exhausted after both events. Lupus was active again. I started to feel sick around December 28, 2012.

Battle No. 5

In less than a year, I got sick again! This time, I came directly to New York City and stayed for a while. I lived with my daughter and family in New York City. Luckily, I was granted disability which included health insurance. This has been a blessing. I was not admitted but my doctors took good care of me at Mount Sinai. I got my medications and follow what the doctor ordered. Since I have decided to stay in New York for a while and take care of my health, I started to think about things I could engage myself with to keep me busy while I am in New York. I would like to engage in consultancy in education for different organizations in Sierra Leone and the USA, especially universities around New York City. I have done some consultancies with schools, colleges, and business organizations in Sierra Leone. I did extensive consultancy with the Environmental and Protection Agency of Sierra Leone (EPA-SL) where I established environmental clubs to be used as vehicles to implement environmental programs in homes, schools, and communities. So I thought it would be nice to do some work in education and I enjoyed it too. I also represented EPA-SL on national and international forum at the United Nations in New York City. Reports were produced and forwarded to EPA-SL. I attended local EPA-SL meeting where I represented the organization. Mainly, I engaged in short-term work to engage my time while I am recuperating from my illness. New York City is becoming my new home away from Sierra Leone slowly. Besides, I have established a great medical team with Mount Sinai and I feel good about staying in New York City. Additionally, the city has a great transportation system that made life easier for me.

As soon as I felt better again, I had the urge to go back to Sierra Leone. Around December 2013, I decided that I will give

Sierra Leone another chance. So I packed my stuff and left again. Also, during the winter, I like to go somewhere warm. Sierra Leone seems to be an easier option for me. This way, I get to see family and get to spend time with my mom. I arrived in Sierra Leone happily and had a very good festive Christmas holiday. I enjoyed the time with family and especially with our mom. She enjoys singing and when we are around her, she always sings and tell stories. I also kept myself busy engaging with short projects with EPA working with Environmental Nature Clubs in schools and colleges. At this time, I had ceased my employment with the USL. I really could not do full-time work anymore. My health has gotten very challenging. I was also busy with a building construction for a home in Sierra Leone. My daughter, her husband, and I are developing it together.

On February 24, 2014, I turned fifty years old. It was a great time for me. My daughter, Malik, and Dr. Julie Goodwin came to Sierra Leone to celebrate with me. I was especially delighted to have my grandson around. Their visits made my birthday very fun and extra special. It was a blessing to have them over. On the day of my birthday, I was treated to a scrumptious lunch at one of my favorite eatery in Sierra Leone, Florence. Florence is an Italian seafood restaurant that is located on one of the many beachfronts in Sierra Leone. It was beautiful and had lunch on that day with Namina, my niece, Leeann, Julie, and Malik. We had a great time. The following Sunday, I celebrated my birthday with a church service followed by lunch at Freetown Lumley Beach and at one of my favorite hangout spot, Wazobia. First we went to church for a thanksgiving service and ended up at the beach where lunch was served. We danced till later in the evening.

During this same period, the Ebola virus surfaced in neighboring Guinea and Liberia. We were very scared it will come to Sierra Leone. Dr. Goodwin, my daughter, and grandson departed for the United States in early March 2014.

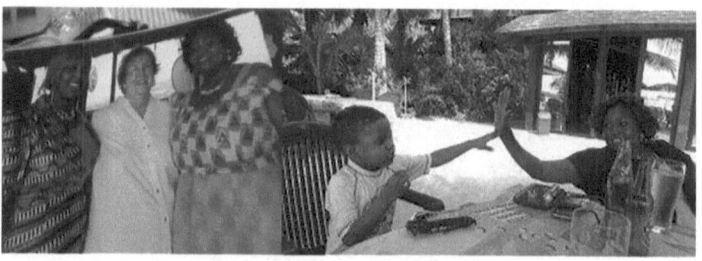

Birthday Celebration Pictures: Leeann,
Julie and I, and Malik and I

Battle No. 6

I had plans to return back to the United States in October
but due to the Ebola virus in Sierra Leone, Liberia, Guinea, and
considering my health situation; I decided to return to New York
the soonest. Besides, I got sick and I was admitted at Choithram
Hospital at Hill Station in Freetown. During my three-day stay at
Choitharam, it seems people died every minute. It was traumatizing
and I thought I was next on the list to die. My niece, Dr. Fatu Forna
Sesay and husband, Dr. Sheku Sesay, who are both doctors in Atlanta
were in Sierra Leone on a medical mission and they visited me at the
hospital. They strongly recommended that I go to the United States
immediately. Between, my oldest sister, Ebun, and her husband, Mr.
Robert Strassser King, we arranged for my plane ticket expeditiously
and I was on my way to New York City on the next available flight.
Upon arrival in New York City, my daughter and husband picked me
up from the airport and I was whisked to Mount Sinai ER. Because
Ebola was rampant in Sierra Leone as well as it was in neighboring
countries and highly contagious, I was quarantined so they would
rule out Ebola. It was scary to see people in yellow medical gowns
and masks to come see me as it reminded me of the Ebola situation
back home. Center for Disease Control (CDC) was alerted and they
came to Mount Sinai to ensure they were ready to handle the situation if it was an Ebola case. I mean, they meant business, and they
were very diligent! It was impressive! If the medical system worked

like what I experienced at Mount Sinai, folks will not die so easily and Ebola would have no chance! Thankfully, it was concluded that I did not have Ebola. However my immune system was weak and it seems I was facing a bout of lupus again. I was informed that I was very lucky this time, if I had waited any longer, my immune system would have shut down and it would have been difficult to save my life. I was very scared! I was admitted for about a week and discharged. Let me tell you, the stigmatization regarding Ebola and people from the continent of Africa during the outbreak was a huge problem globally. People were very hostile toward Africans as they were scared of the virus and thought Africans owned the virus. I was so scared that I refused to wear my African clothes and to say I am African. One time at a McDonald's, my daughter caught me lying to someone who said, "I love your accent, where is it from?" and I replied "the Virgin Islands!" Leeann told me that I don't have to lie and not everyone will stigmatize Africans. For some reason I was very paranoid!

By July 2014, the Ebola outbreak had taken over Sierra Leone. I was scared for my family including my mom. My eldest sister, Ebun, was in Sierra Leone at the time and she handled the situation and ensured that the family was safe. Thankfully, we did not suffer any loss of immediate family members from the epidemic. My family followed the rules of CDC and World Health Organization's (WHO) rules and regulations. This battle with Ebola lasted for more than a year in that region of West Africa. It made it difficult for anyone to return to Sierra Leone. I stayed in the United States for the rest of the year and kept myself busy looking for consultancies. I applied for short-term work at Columbia and NYU as well to get myself ready for substitute teaching in schools. One of my former students at FBC, who was studying in Japan, linked me up with an opportunity in his university in Japan. I was lucky to write a paper that was accepted at the university for a presentation. I wrote on Ebola in Sierra Leone. All expenses were paid and a stipend was offered to me as well. It was an amazing experience. I am very thankful to one of my former student, Mr. Abu Bakarr Jalloh, from Fourah Bay College (FBC) who made it possible for me to have that opportunity. I spent one week in Japan and came back. I had a great time, but I was looking forward to coming back to America and eventually going back to Sierra Leone. No place like home with family.

This was my first winter in New York City, and it was not easy. It was very cold! When it's cold, my bones hurt, and my breathing is very challenging due to the lupus. Very cold weather is not friendly with lupus and interstitial lungs disease. Anyway, I weathered the storm and stayed indoors a lot. Nowadays I am much accustomed to the change in weather and mind ready so I handle it better. If I can, I still like to go visit somewhere warm in the winter. Sierra Leone was not a safe place for anyone that year due to the Ebola epidemic so I had to live with the cold. It wasn't that bad after all.

My rheumatoid nodules were getting bigger and painful each day, making it impossible to use my right arm. I was referred to an arm orthopedic doctor at Mount Sinai. He examined my hand, did MRI, X-ray, and scan. He told me it's nodules and it could be done through a complex-but-easy surgery. He could remove it, he said. So we scheduled a date for the surgery. I figured I could do it in the winter since I will be home most of the time. It was two hours or so surgery, and painful. It took a long time to heal. For about two months or so, I was unable to utilize my right arm. So, writing, typing, lifting, and hair braiding, which I enjoyed, had to stop. I managed to cook and do light work.

Around March 2015, I went to Gambia to visit my sister Ade, who was the head of UN in the Gambia. I also networked with universities and schools there to see how we could bring CAPS to the Gambia but it did not work out. I was able to meet with schools, the university, government officials, and other officials. In fact, I did some presentations at some of the schools and the university as well. It was great networking but not fruitful and my health could not permit me as well. It was a very pleasant trip, and I had a great time. I also visited Ghana. Some good friends of mine who I met in Tallahassee retired and moved back to Ghana. I visited them and it was awesome to spend time with them. I visited universities there as well for possible consultancy but not fruitful either. It was a great reunion for us and I had a great time. I was sad because I was not able to visit Sierra Leone due to Ebola. My feet were itching to go to Sierra Leone, but it was not safe. Also, I missed my mom as I haven't seen her in a while. After a couple of weeks, I returned back to the United States.

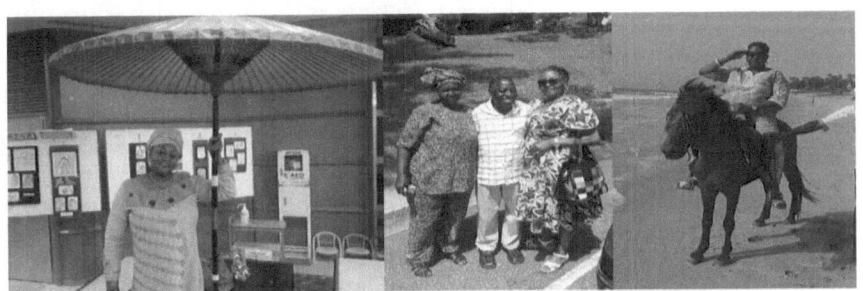

Japan (me) Ghana (Dr. and Mrs. Owusu and I) me in Gambia

The Ebola virus rampaged Sierra Leone, Liberia, and Guinea. The epidemic killed more than five thousand people in less than two years. Life came to a standstill in these three countries. Education stopped, and businesses were closed. There was a major health crisis. Starvation was on the rise, and many of the prominent and good medical personnel were killed by the virus. It took the whole world to save these countries. Everyone had to contribute. Doctors and medical experts came to the aid of these countries from every parts of the world. It took them more than a year to win the battle with Ebola. If the world hadn't stepped in, it could have become a global virus. Luckily they did, and it was eradicated in these countries. These three countries were set back decades behind development by the outbreak. They were already impoverishing states, but after Ebola, they got worse. The Ebola crises just quadrupled the problems of the country. Sierra Leone and Liberia who just recovered from more than ten years of civil war suffered more damages. Infrastructures, medical, and development were distorted. By October 2015, the region was free of the virus. At this time I was itchy to go to Sierra Leone and I missed my mom very much.

So on October 31, 2015, I boarded Brussels Airlines to go to Sierra Leone. I landed in Sierra Leone on November 1, 2015. I was full of joy, and the first person I saw at home was my sweet mama. I was excited! I hugged her and we talked for a long time. We shared a bed and kept each other's company daily and nightly. My other sister, Remi, who is the fourth born was with our mom all the time came along. All three of us spent valuable time together. In fact, she is her caretaker, may God bless her. Our mom ordered her around and bossed her around all the time due to old-age crisis that was due to circumstances beyond her control. I mean, she loved her Remie and wouldn't want to hurt her at all. But Remi was always gentle, sweet, and mild with mom. When mom moves, she moves, when she shakes, she shakes! I spent time with both my mom and my sister for the whole entire week. We stayed home and enjoyed each other's company. We slept in the same room and we had such great time. Family members came each day to visit and they brought good foods along. It was much-needed celebration.

On November 8, Sunday, I did not attend mass as the weather was stormy and bad to drive. So I stayed home with mom and my sister. Family members came by and we prepared scrumptious meals. I had a special friend who stood by my side all this time. He is the great Lamdi. Even though he didn't have much to give, I can always count on his support and compassion. One night, I had to be rushed to Choithram Hospital and he was right there with my sister's husband to take me to the hospital. Lamdi was one I could count on. We had a great Sunday with mom at home, just relaxing. We played games, told jokes, and had a pleasant day on Sunday, November 8, 2015. I remembered there was no singing! Mom asked me to take a ride with her in the car but the weather was just bad and it rained the heaviest that I ever seen in November in Freetown. We watched movies and kept each other's company. We had supper. My mother loves bread, butter, a cup of tea with milk and sugar. She had that and said good night. We took her to bed. By 1:30 a.m. on Monday, November 9, 2015, my mother was gone! She slipped off in her sleep! That was the end of our sweet mother. May her gentle soul rest in perfect peace! I will never forget her as she was an amazing mother who worked tirelessly!

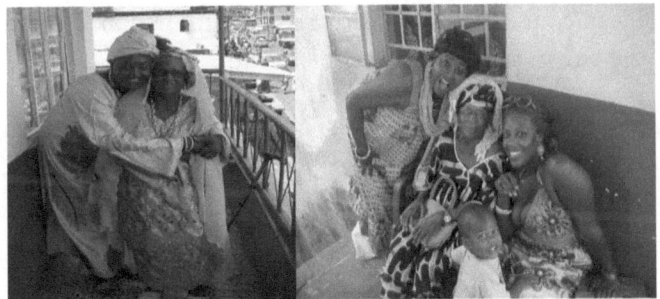

Mom and I   Mom, Me, Leeann, and Malik

It was a sad day! I tried to wake her up but she was gone to heaven and never to return. She calls it the one-way travel/trip without a return! We had to call families to inform them one by one. By the morning, the house was full with families and friends. A few days later the foundation of my life was laid to rest at the Kissy Mess Mess Cemetery. That is the end of a great chapter in my life and my hero was gone!

After the funeral our oldest sister, who is in politics, just got assigned to serve as the Ambassador to Senegal. In early January, she packed and moved away to Dakar. Both the third and fourth born moved away from Sierra Leone at the same time as well. Now I am the only sibling remaining in Sierra Leone. Without Mama and my sisters, it was hard living in Sierra Leone. I felt empty! Although I had great support but I miss their presence. I had plans to return to the United States in March. However, I got sick in February and I had to be rushed to New York. As soon as I arrived in New York City, I was whisked to the ER. I was treated for a stomach infection and was admitted for about one week. Leeann's husband Pateh, Leeann, and Malik were with me and they were worried about me. Malik was so scared that he begged the doctor to please don't let her grandma die. The doctor took him very serious and whispered in my ears, you will be well soon, I assured your grandson of that! I went home after a week of hospital stay. But I was still feeling sick. So I visited my doctors many times complaining that I was not feeling well. My breathing was extremely off. I was feeling like I needed help to breathe. They kept increasing and decreasing my prednisone and I was not getting better. Since lupus is a disease to be managed, I continued to weather the storm and prayed to feel better.

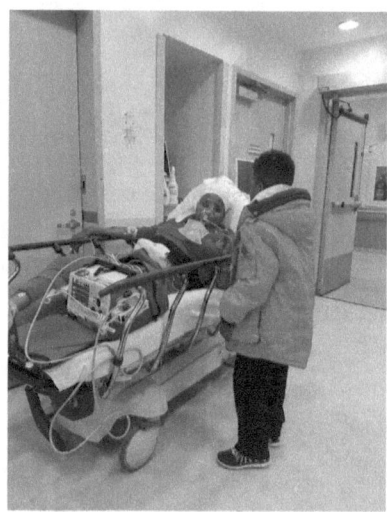

Malik looking over me

Battle No. 7

I was feeling better again. Julie, my friend, and I planned a girls' trip. We were heading for Florida, Texas, and California. On the first leg of our trip to Florida, we ended in Tallahassee. Julie got sick and she was hospitalized. She has health issues and aging was taking a toll on her life as well. Although we are good friends, she is much older than me, but she has a youthful heart. We get along very well. Unfortunately, her daughters had to make the call and flew her back to Albany, New York. I continued my journey to Dallas, Texas, hoping to finish our trip and tell Julie all about it. In Texas, I began to feel ill. My breathing was off and I had heavy pain when I breathe. My nephew, Donald Taylor, took me to the Makene Hospital ER. I was admitted for pneumonia. I stayed there for a week. During my admittance, they overloaded me with prednisone. I was too weak that I wasn't sure of the dosage of prednisone I was given at the time.

It was when I started feeling very bad and my sugar levels were plunging to an alarming low numbers that I questioned my medications. For some strange reason, my sugar level was dropping drastically. One night I was so sick and my sugar dropped to level number 29. Normal sugar range is 80–120. So 29 was very low and almost coma status. They had to inject sugar into my stomach for the very first time to prevent me in going into a coma. I was released from the hospital after a week. I was given sugar testing equipment to monitor my sugar levels. I had to eat sweets to ensure that my sugar levels are not low. It was rough and I ballooned up. As soon as I was released from the hospital, I rested in Dallas with my sister for a week. Then I ended my trip and came to New York City.

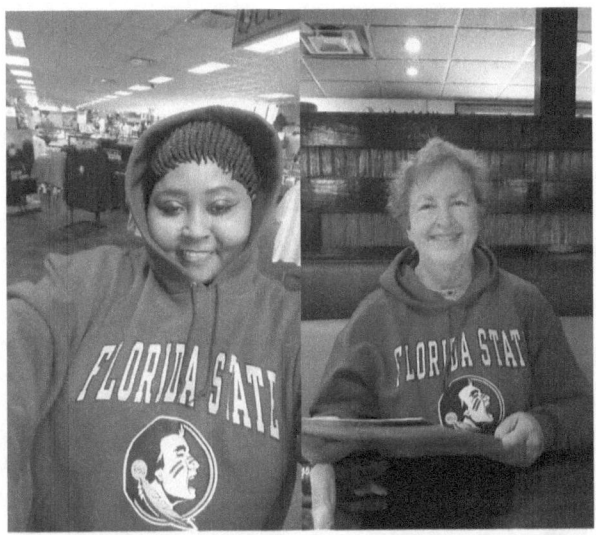

Visiting our Alma Mater, Florida State University

As soon as I arrived in New York, I went to see my doctors, and I complained about my lung pain especially when I breathe. I had some coughing and the coughing got worse. I saw them several times and they thought it could be cold or bronchitis. I was treated for these symptoms and I continue to feel bad. One early morning in early March, I felt like I could not breathe and my lungs were gone. My daughter, her husband, a friend who was visiting me, and Malik all got very worried for me and they called 911. The ambulance came and picked me up. They wanted to take me to Harlem Hospital but I pleaded with them that they take me to Mount Sinai as all my doctors are located there and I prefer to go there. I was taken to Mount Sinai Hospital. At Mount Sinai, the illness continues and my breathing was really off and very painful when I breathe as well as when I cough. I could not sleep, I could not eat and continue to feel sick. I cried all night, and most of the time, I had sleepless nights. My appetite was very poor. I was placed on oxygen on 24-7! I needed help to even breathe. I beg them to please help me. My sugar was low, my appetite was poor, I had sleepless nights, and my breathing was very off and painful with a lot of coughing. I have been in Mount Sinai for about two weeks, and I am still feeling sick. I insisted they do further testing on me to help me please. I mean they had to work on my low sugar levels, breathing problem, lupus, and lung issues along with the cough. I insisted and persisted that I was not well and something must be done. My medical team had meetings upon meetings with me at week two in the hospital. Since my coughing was persistent and affecting my breathing we agreed to tackle that problem first, then the sugar and any other problems later on.

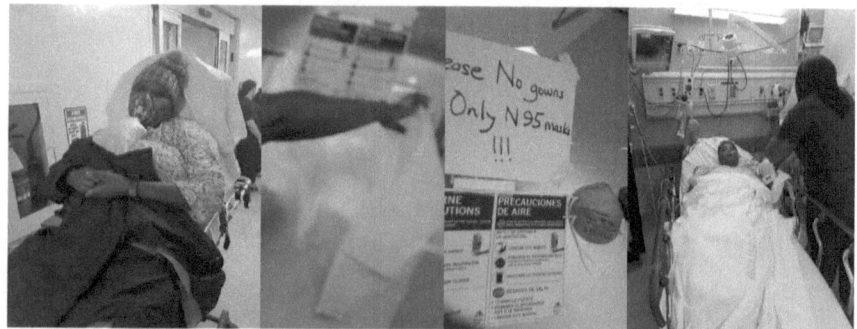

Pictures of Me at Mount Sinai Where I Was Admitted

For the breathing and coughing, I had X-rays done, blood works, spittle test to check for any lung infection and all came back negative. I was still coughing and hurting still. But the X-ray showed some round sport in my lungs that look like pneumonia. So they treated me with antibiotics but the pain still continues and so was the coughing. The CDC was informed of my situation and they visited me at the hospital. They decided to do a bronchial test where a tube was passed down my lungs to get to the spot so they could do a biopsy and test it further. A day later I was taken for the surgery. It took three days to get the results of the test result. On the third day after the surgical procedure, the medical team came to my room and broke the horrible news that they found tuberculosis (TB) down my lungs. I cried so hard and did not want to believe it! They immediately provided the treatment plan to me. It included six more weeks in the hospital in isolation because the disease is airborne. Additionally, I had to take about a dozen medications each day plus my lupus medications. They added that I have to take the TB medications for a minimum of six months. Also, they informed me that I will receive a call from the New York Health Department in regards to the TB. Since TB is a public health issue as it is airborne, the government has to be informed. I received a call from the health department and they visited me right away. I was informed that it is serious and I must follow-through with all treatment or they would isolate me for all the treatment. Also they demanded all my family contact and they followed up with appointments to get them tested for TB. I thought I was going crazy! I was hysterical, nervous, in denial, and heartbroken. They had a big sign in my room that anyone who enters must wear a mask. I was allowed to walk around with mask on my floor. Sometimes, I see nurses walk around with the yellow gowns as well and a mask. That got me scared as Ebola was fresh in my mind with the Sierra Leone Ebola crisis. I could just imagine the nurses, doctors, and all medical personnel with the yellow gowns during the times of Ebola in Africa. I didn't like the sight of it at all. I prayed very hard each day. I prayed for strength and courage to get over this point in my life. I felt like I was in jail or something similar. I cannot begin to tell you how I felt about it, I was in misery. My daughter, my son-in-law, and Malik were constantly visiting. I don't know what it would have been like without them. Also, some of my daughter's friends and my son-in-law's relatives visited me as well. A few friends of mine came to see me as well. To God be the glory and praising him, I was able to go through this unimaginable time. As a catholic, I said the rosary each day. It strengthens my faith in Christ. Also, the catholic ministries of Mount Sinai visited every Sunday and sometimes during the week. My TB treatments continued at the hospital.

The very sad thing about this whole experience is that my whole family was subjected to TB tests! I was scared that they would have TB. I was scared especially for Malik as we were very close and he slept on my bed several times. Just the thought that he might have it drove me crazy! I prayed that they didn't have it. By God's grace and miraculously they were all negative. How I got the infection, I couldn't tell you. I know it is very prevalent in Sierra Leone. The fact that lupus has weakened my immune system, makes me vulnerable to catching viruses, infections, and/or diseases. Also, because of my lung disease, I could get pulmonary infections easily. In fact, I had gotten pneumonia and bronchitis several times.

I was constantly given medications to bring my sugar levels to normal range (between 70 mg/dL and 120 mg/dL [3.8 and 5.5 mmol]) as it kept going lower than the normal range. Because low blood sugar is dangerous and could be fatal, it is important to monitor one's sugar level at all times. When my sugar is low, I could easily tell as I feel weak and could hardly do anything. I couldn't even sleep. I mean everything that needs energy in the body is impacted. Because sugar gives the body energy and when the body doesn't have enough of it, it basically cannot function well. Every movement in the body needs oxygen. When my sugar gets low, I could not even control my urination or even blink my eyes. I felt like I was in some kind of a trance and it was very challenging!

After six weeks of the TB treatment at the hospital, they removed the isolation label from my room. I no longer wore masks and neither did my visitors. In regards to my sugar, they suspect that I may have insulinoma. Insulinomas are small tumors that are found in the pancreas. Because they are tiny it is hard to find them. The only way to find insulinomas is to search for them in the pancreas very carefully. So a surgical procedure was ordered to go into my pancreas to look for insulinoma. While sedated they went into my pancreas with a microscopic camera that they used to look for the tumors. Thankfully, they did not find any tumors in my pancreas. So the research on my sugar levels continued. After about nine weeks at Mount Sinai Hospital I was discharged. The plan is to follow up with endocrinologists to follow up on my sugar issues, follow up with pulmonology and rheumatologists, and most importantly to continue with my TB treatment. I also had a sugar testing devise to check my sugar levels. I had to carry snacks with me to help boost my sugar levels as well. I have to continue this until I could see an endocrinologist. Finally I was able to see one. My blood sugar was low that morning and my previous sugar level tests history showed they have been low as well. The endocrinologist asked me for my list of medication, and I shared the list with her. She realized I have been using Plaquenil, which is for my lupus. She informed me that she read on some research that long-term use of Plaquenil could cause low sugar problems. She advised that they switched that medication for me. It was switched to CellCept, which has its pros and cons and this is the case for most medications. If they cure you, they cause some other issues as well. I stopped the Plaquenil instantly and to my biggest relief, my sugar problems subsided a great deal. I still have problems but I learnt to manage it. I continued with the TB medications. I had to visit the State Health Department Clinic once a month to follow up with my TB medical updates and test to see if the medications were working. Also, every day I take the TB medications, I had to be videotaped. They have to confirm that I was indeed taking the medications. At this point, I may have done about five months of treatment. All of a sudden they informed me that my TB virus was working against one of the medications and they have to change it to another medication. With the new dose, I may have to be on the TB medication for another year. It was rough, but I made it! After a whole year of visits to the health department and taking my TB medications faithfully, I was given a certificate that states that I was TB free. I felt a huge sense of relief and gave praises to God. After this medical treatment I can breathe better and feel very well!

Next appointment was with my pulmonary doctor. I went for my follow-up visit with him. He sent me for a test to check my oxygen level at rest, at walk, and doing exercise. When walking my oxygen level drops and they determined that I need two liters of oxygen when walking. So they ordered an oxygen concentrator tank for me to keep at home. Then I was given portable ones. However the portables were very heavy to carry and it was difficult to carry them around. Unfortunately, the vendor refused to give smaller ones as they claim my insurance didn't cover smaller ones. I stayed with them for a whole year and once the contract expired, I switched to a vendor that would provide me with lighter portable bottles. It seems like carrying a little oxygen tank is a way of life for me now moving forward. I also needed a nebulizer and inhalers to help with my breathing problems. So far, I am managing my lung issues very well and the pain from breathing has decreased a whole lot. Next was to follow up with my rheumatologist. My rheumatologist advised that I continue with a low dose of prednisone and CellCept. Ibuprofen and Prilosec were taken only when needed for heartburns and pains. Otherwise, my lupus is pretty stable.

All of a sudden, I started to get sharp pains in my big toes and on the swelling on my arm. My toes hurt so bad that I could hardly walk. After some tests, I was informed that I have gout! Gout, what is gout? I really dread any complications. As if I haven't been through enough! *Long* story short, when one has excess uric acid in your toes, it crystalizes and they hurt. That is basically gout. I got some medications for it and it has helped. I later found out that the gout came from some of the TB medications. I have found with lupus medications and many other medications, if they cure something they might leave something or create a side effect.

Next, I had to deal with the swollen arm. I was informed that they are linked to lupus as they are a form of arthritis. I was referred to orthopedics for further diagnostics. They did X-ray and MRI. It was determined that they may need to remove the rheumatoid nodules to relieve me of my pain. They also found that I have some carpal tunnel syndrome issues as well. The nodules were becoming painful and unbearable as well as getting huge. A surgical procedure was recommended. It took two surgeries to really give me the relief I needed in my arm. After the surgeries, it's a bit swollen, but I praise

God that the pain has subsided. I am able to now use my hand without pain.

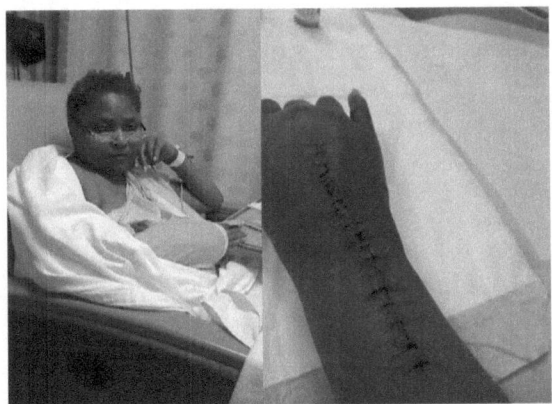

Before and After Surgery

Since I am in charge of my lupus and following doctors' advices, I am feeling better. The battles have seized for now. I pray many a time that lupus disappears or go into remission. In June, I felt heavy breathing issues. I was scared as they were similar to what I felt before I got admitted to the hospital. I don't like to bother my daughter about my illness or even bother my family or anyone regarding my illness. So I took myself to the Mount Sinai ER. I was breathing really badly and I got even more worried. Upon arrival at the hospital, I was immediately placed on oxygen. My sugar levels were low and they had to take care of that first. My chest was X-rayed and they found out that I have pneumonia again. The sad thing is that I had to be admitted at the hospital. I cried and I was confused! The medical folks were confused and I told them that I am frightened because I came to the hospital like this the last and I ended up staying for more than two months. I didn't want that to happen to me again. I didn't want to stay in the hospital but didn't have a choice. The doctor said they needed to monitor me for at least a night. I settled down and called Leeann. I informed her that I was in the hospital and I was admitted for pneumonia again. I cried and she consoled me. She and Malik visited me later that evening. I did let a few of my sisters know as well. In two days, I felt better and I was discharged. I came home with a huge relief and was very happy! Since the June 2018 bout, I am staying pretty well. But some of the aches and difficulties breathing along with some sugar issues are still challenges. My God is in control and I look up to him. I am thankful for an awesome family and friends.

4

Putting the Pieces of My
Lupus Puzzle Together

What is really lupus to me and why I think I got it?

I introduced lupus a bit at the onset of this book. However, the more I live with it, the more I get to understand it more and do further research about it so I could get a good grip of it. I found that lupus is systemic lupus erythematosus (SLE), which is an autoimmune disease. This means that the body's immune system mistakenly attacks healthy tissue and organs. Lupus may lead to long-term inflammation, swelling, pain, and damage that can affect many different body systems, including the heart, lungs, brain, kidneys, joints, and skin. Since the symptoms of lupus are similar to other diseases including periods of illness or "flares" and periods of feeling fine or "remission," it can be tricky to diagnose. It's not contagious and it is not related to cancer. The exact cause is not known, it is believed that it results from a mix of genetics and the person's environment. Experts believe that people with a genetic predisposition to the disease may develop lupus when something in their environment triggers it. Triggers include certain medicines, certain chemicals, tobacco smoke, infections, sun exposure, and a very stressful life. Currently, there is no known cure but people with lupus are given treatments to help manage its symptoms. Approximately 1.5 million Americans have it, and it is more common in women than men, typically striking in the childbearing years (ages fifteen to forty-four).

I believe that I had a predisposition to Lupus from my family heritage somewhere. I often think it's from my dad, as I watched him go through several ailments in his later years. He seemed tired most of the time. He had worked super hard as a young man. Plus, he must have had a very stressful life living a polygamous life with several children. Because he worked very hard and saved up money, retiring early was not so bad for him. He had many houses and had saved some money as well. He also had several wives and several children who were at his beck and call. Although he was set for a nice retirement, he went through many stresses as well. So he may have been predisposed to lupus too. However, he was never diagnosed and lupus is tricky to be pinpointed. It takes several advance medical tests to determine that one has lupus. I feel blessed and lucky to have been in the USA and my lupus was caught early. So I feel that I may have inherited lupus from a family member, but I couldn't really tell as members of my families were never diagnosed.

I also feel strongly that my environment overtime played a key role in breaking my immune system down. I was sexually, physically, and mentally abused as a young girl. I didn't feel like I have any place to run to or anyone to talk to and this was common for most children during my time in Sierra Leone. I dealt with it all alone most of the time. As an adult, I read that bed-wetting is related to child sexual abuse. When I was a little girl, I wet the bed many times. When I woke up in the morning, family members including my mother would shame me publicly for wetting the bed and sometimes gave me public flogging. The whole community knew that I am a bed-wetter. People feel that shaming and public flogging is a cure for bed-wetting behavior as it may cause the victims to stop bed-wetting. Also, I was always scared and afraid of the dark. In fact, my siblings will frighten me that the big fat man was coming to get me, and I would scream and beg them not to leave me alone. I lived in shame and fear as well as a very insecure childhood life. Sometimes, I felt so alone that I prayed for God to take my life away. As a child, I would have easily committed suicide if I only knew how. I was in constant fear and shame. Children were quick to get molested when I was growing up in Sierra Leone and the community or relatives fail to see it through the eyes of the child. Although I don't blame the communities or families as they didn't know any better either. In retrospect, many young girls and boys around my age, who were bed-wetting or very much afraid may have been trying to tell something to the adults around them. Adults would dismiss these behaviors or reprimand the children because they were ignorant of the meaning of the behaviors. Even when I was bullied at school or by anyone, I was quiet and I will not say a damn word most of the time for fear that I will get bullied and called names by my peers and I hated the name calling as well. I remembered the first time I fought back at school. My mom went ballistic on me for fighting. I was tired of being bullied and I decided to fight back. My uniforms were torn in every angle and I did give out some whipping that day that some of the bullies ran away. In fact they went and told on me to my mom. When I got home, I was in pain. Mom gave me a good licking! Since that day, I gained some respect among my peers and the bullying ceased a bit. Now that they know I could fight back and actually whip some asses too. I was determined to fight and irrespective of the outcome at home and that is exactly what happened.

My stepmother was fond of giving provoking names to children. She called me "Lazyloss." She thought I was too lazy and don't want to work at all. Because I was lazy, I gained all the laziness of the world. So, if you feel like your laziness is missing, Lola has it! I hated that name up till now. When she tries to call me out, she would say lazy loss and I was supposed to say, "Yes, Ma." If and when I don't answer, I will get a whipping. She would tease me and even ask me, "My lazy is missing, and who found it?" I would say, "I did" or "Lola found it!" That was how she would want me to answer. I used to despise the torture and mental abuse. At an older age, she tried to call me that. Thank God I stood up against it! I flipped on her and I told her never to call me that again. I told her that I may have been lazy in her book or mind, when I was little and only a child. Now, I am older, wiser, a college graduate, a mother, a homeowner, and I have a full-time job. That is not how lazy people behave and she must never call me that name again. At first she was sarcastic about it. Thankfully she hasn't called me that ever since. She had demeaning names for everyone and even her own biological children. She even have other names for me. For some reasons, giving me funny silly names was something she enjoyed and it made me feel sick to my stomach as a small child. One time she called one of her children, "Omolanke!" Omalanke is wagon-type mechanism that is pushed around in Sierra Leone for delivery. Her child did not do well in school and she received an assisted promotion to a new class. So my stepmother called her Omolanke, that is to mean that she was pushed to a new grade and not promoted by her hard work! She despised it and the look on her face was defeating! But that was the work of her biological mother, who am I to butt in? These names have negative lasting impacts on young people. A very sad one case that I blamed my stepmother and my dad for is a name given to one of my half-brothers. He is the biological son of my stepmother. Apparently, the boy was conceived from another man and not of my dad's. They named him Jebu. Jebu in the Yoruba tribe of Nigeria where my dad hails from means counterfeit, fake, or not authentic! Imagine carrying such a name with you all your life. You have to live with the fact that you were born to another man while your mother was married to another man then deal with that name as well. It is stigmatizing! I tell you, that young man hasn't done much for himself up till now. I am certain that his birth situation plus his name given to him has placed him in a confused state of mind up till today. He seems confused and doesn't really know where he is heading. He is married to a strong woman, who works very hard. They have very smart and intelligent children, but the dad is not strong as a dad for them. He is hopeless at times. I have come to his family's rescue a lot but it is a difficult situation, especially factoring the economic state of Sierra Leone.

As an adult, I always burst my behind in whatever I signed up for just to prove to my stepmother and the world that I was not a "Lazyloss." I went through many educations including vocational schools and worked many jobs to prove to myself that I am not a Lazyloss type, at least not now! I did this unconsciously but it's true. I worked tirelessly like my dad. Some people in Tallahassee have asked me what I was proving that I had to work so hard and gather so many certificates! I have a certificate in childcare, clerical accounting, cosmetology and facial beauty, nail technology, associate's degree, Bachelor of Science, and a master's degree! One of my African American friends asked if I wanted to take all the educations in America to Africa! I laughed at her sarcasm as she was joking but I answered and told her that I came a long way from Sierra Leone and I wanted to make my folks proud. Honestly, if it wasn't because of lupus, I would have been in a PhD Program by now. But who knows, it may happen either in an honorary way or actual work! I often think that this overworked attitude may have contributed to some of my environmental stress that brought on lupus.

The mental abuse and physical abuse that is associated with FGM, childminding, early marriage, and other stressors may have also contributed largely as to why lupus crept up upon me. As a child, for the most part I lived with my parents or mother. My dad had families in Nigeria and Sierra Leone so he spent his time juggling between Nigeria and Sierra Leone. At some time of my life, I lived with my older sister and I lived with an elderly well-respected lady in the community as well. I called these my childminding days!

Growing up with my parents was OK and I felt safe most of the time. Young girls in my immediate family were sexually molested by families and friends who visited. Also, our house was a community-type living compound. My mother rented parts of the house to people. Some of these folks were sexually abusive to young girls around. There were two prominent pedophiles living in our compound and my mother and other adults didn't even know of them. Their victims were scared to speak out, including me.

At the elderly lady's house, I was subjected to slave type of lifestyles. I was about fourteen years old. I did all her laundry, cooked her meals, ran all her market errands, cleaned her house, and so much more. I was exhausted and tired most of the time. My eldest sister thought that it would strengthen me and help me out academically as the lady was a famous teacher and she might help me with my school stuff. Instead, I received mental and physical abuse. Because I wet the bed, she made me sleep on cold floors. Because of this, I had my first episode with pneumonia at about age fourteen. I was admitted and had to be treated for two weeks. I ran away from the hospital because I was scared of the shots and just afraid, period! I was given shots every day and I simply couldn't handle it no more. Also, I was sexually molested there as well. The old lady's house was too much for me so I ran away. Honestly, it was a very negative experience living there and I really did not benefit from living with her academically at all. I was miserable, tired, and I had no time to do my school work. I still blame my sister for that but she doesn't seem to recall that situation. My elder sister is like the matriarch. So whatever she says holds water when we were little and my mother went with the flow. I often think that environment may have contributed to how my immune started to quench!

At my elder sister's all the children worked hard and it wasn't so bad. As all of us know that is what is expected of us. But my brother in law, my sister's husband was kind of strict and we thought he was evil at times. We were scared to even mention his name. We have the feeling that he will hear us. So, we made up a name for him and we used that name instead of his real name. We called him "Gaba the short form of Gerbazon!" That was the name given to one of the toughest villains in old Indian movies. He was like a father figure to all of us as well. Well, he told me that upon our father's passing away, our father had asked him to take care of his family as he was not sure of when he will return back to Freetown. My dad was from Nigeria and he was heading back to Nigeria due to health issues. I was able to stay at his house and enjoy my teenage life because there were young girls and boys my age there. We kept each other's company and played with each other. But sexual molestation prey that house! Many a time, I have to fight to save myself from the evils of young men living in the house or just visiting. Gaba was a politician and a womanizer as well. Also, he was a wealthy man during that time. He had a tennis court in his compound so different distinguished folks come there to play. As a politician, his house catered for visitors that came through all the time and sometimes they spend the night. When they do come around, they prey on the young girls around. Even the other young boys who lived in the house have tried sexual encounters with me and other young girls several times. It was a war to fight for your body at that house. God really saved me. But there were many young girls who were unlucky in that house.

I am not sure if my sister or her husband knew about it. As kids we were thought to shut up and simply be quiet! This environment was good to live in only if you know how to survive and fight to save your body. I was getting good at that and I tried hard. But it was very stressful, and I could see how it may have impacted lupus in some ways. Also, there were so many inside fighting, physical and emotional abuse amidst the sexual harassments. It was like the land of the survival of the fittest indeed!

FGM is one pain that I never forget. Up till now my heart throbs when I think of it. I really didn't know the depth of what was going to happen to me. I suspected it has to do with my private body parts but I didn't realize that my clitoris and labia will be completely removed by using a razor blade! As I write, I had to take a break and pray. It was the most painful and traumatic experience I ever experienced. If someone had schooled me about it, trust me I would not have gone through such a barbaric trauma. I despise it! For the first time in my life, I felt hatred toward my mom as I felt that she knew about the pain and she let me go through it. She apologized and told me that it was her culture and they kind of forced her to have her girls initiated. She felt helpless and had to follow and respect her tradition. This group has some powers, I tell you. It is hard to defeat them but if I could get my late mom to give them up, I am sure the day will come when FGM will be history. My dad did not really like the idea but he was defeated by my mother and her clans. FGM added to my insecurities of life and even doubled my insecurities upon arrival in the USA. All of a sudden you become educated on issues and realized that your own people mutilated you and robbed you of God's gift of pleasure. Sad! The pain of the thought of FGM is always depressing and stressful!

Another sad element of FGM was when my baby sister was mutilated right in front of me and I couldn't help her. She was screaming and fighting but I had just been mutilated so I couldn't help her as I was in pain and I could hardly move. It was disgusting! I felt like those women were like godlike figure and I depend on them or they might cut off other parts of our bodies. I mean we are at their mercy! FGM is very painful and horrible. The day after the mutilation, trying to urinate was the most painful experience. It hurts so bad that I refused to urinate. I wouldn't drink either. Because I didn't urinate for days, the lips area matted up! It's even more difficult to urinate now. So the lady in charge of checking came to check to see if I was healing well. They realized I had matted up. She called a few other women; they laid me down and physically pulled my vagina area skin apart to open my urethra area. It was very painful and traumatic! FGM created a huge number in my mind and I will never forget it.

At first, I wasn't outspoken as they overwhelmed you with fear during the initiation. They tell you if you ever speak of it, your stomach will swell and burst open and your vagina will go rotten. Some lies and to play with your mind so you don't speak about it. But when I started talking and nothing changed on me, I just continued to expose them. My people believe in voodoo and witchcrafts so they are gullible with statements and they are easy to blackmail. Whenever I meet a boyfriend, who is not familiar with FGM, I have to educate them that I have a missing clitoris and both labia due to my initiation into FGM. I usually have to narrate so much to them. Most of the time, my boyfriends would become sympathetic and scared not to hurt me during sexual intercourse or play. But I tell them to go for it and that it is well and healed! So now it is easier to talk about it. Do I think there is a lupus moment here? I think so, big time!

Last but not the least, is early marriage! Actually this is the finish up and the bigger reason for lupus to come out in me. I really think early marriage triggered and woke up lupus in me finally. I married quite young and moved to Florida from Sierra Leone. I came to join my husband who was a student at FSU at the tender age of eighteen. He was doing his master's and later PhD. My husband was abusive physically, emotionally, and sexually. He actually chastised and physically abused me a few times in Freetown because he saw some guys were holding my hands. I broke up with him several times. He always seems to find people to convince me to forgive him. My very best friend Abi B was one that he used. He would beg her to come and plead his case and that he would never abuse me again. After a while I believed him and gave him chances over and over again.

During our dating, one time he cheated and slept with a girl that he knew. The girl gave him gonorrhea. He found out right away. Before he found out, we had unprotected sex and he knew I would have caught gonorrhea and he knew I had no clue about it. He came crying and explained his predicament and said he wanted to take full responsibility for it. So he has made arrangements for me to see a doctor and get treated. He added that he knows he disrespected our relationship and if I am not interested in him after the incident, that I can do whatever I want. I wished I had left him then. But I was very naive and trusted him even more. He was a young lecturer at the college in Sierra Leone and he was older than me and I admired his honesty. So I started to love and believe in him. I said that I started to love him because at first I had a boyfriend that I loved and Felix tricked me into leaving him so we could be together. He held my head under water so I gave up and broke up with my boyfriend and continued a relationship with Felix. I saw the signs but I ignored them as I was immature and a young girl myself. Plus, I have no one to run to or get advice. We didn't have a support system like that growing up. Anyway, upon my arrival in the United States, I wanted to go to college as well. He thought we could not afford college for the two of us at the same time so I had to wait until he was finished with school. Instead of just working, I went to vocational schools. First, I studied childcare and later I studied clerical accounting. He was very absent at home. He went to school all day and most evenings. He also worked night shifts at the dormitories. I was alone most of the time.

Then Leeann came along in 1985. I was a single parent most of the time. I worked, prepared meals, house work and sometimes school work. I hardly get any help from him. He made sure he told me that we are in this country because of his education and he was not willing to shelf it to accommodate me. It was all about his education. So I said to myself that I wasn't having another child in this condition. Things have to change as it was very difficult for me. While making that decision, I got pregnant again and he said we should abort it.

He said that he was not ready. I know that the conditions with handling Leeann alone were very difficult on me. So we signed up for the abortion and I got it done. This decision, I regret up till now. Not giving Leeann a sibling is regretful! But I thank God for Leeann! The abuse in my marriage continued and my husband disrespected me and cheated on me as well. We separated and divorced. Then we reconciled and remarried. Then we finally divorced! During our marriage, one day he told me if I don't fix my pregnancy situation, he would leave me to find a woman who could give him more children. He wanted more kids. I was disgusted! Having gone through two abortions and one living child with him was not a tasteful statement for me. Hence, I geared my mind for the end. Anyhow, after many battles that I have fought and knocked out in our marriage, this was by far my biggest blow. I divorced him and moved on. He is not in this world today. I pray for the repose of his soul and may God grant him eternal rest. Leeann is a woman now and she is married to Pateh Bah. Pateh embraces my love for him and makes me feel welcome in their home. He calls me mommy too! With pride and joy, I must say I have two children! They have given me one grandson and I have another grandson on the way. We are expecting him in July or August 2018. I am looking forward and I can hardly wait to welcome as well as hold my extra blessing from God.

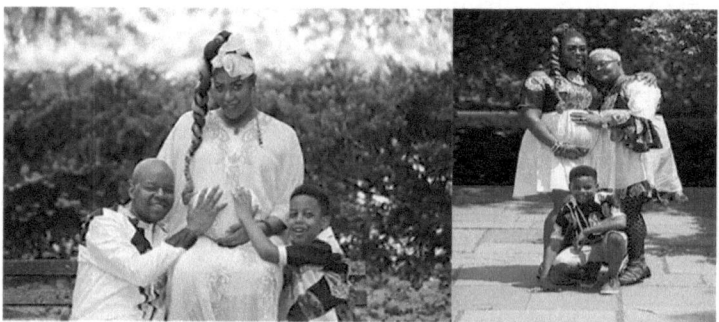

Pateh, Leeann, and Malik   Leeann, Malik, and I

Other Stressors that may have contributed to my lupus situation in my life may have to do with work stress, another marriage, and external factors. I worked for the State of Florida for several years. I always enjoyed my works. Around 1998 a lady was hired to work in our department. She was Caucasian. I trained her to understand the job. She had a bachelor's degree at the time. I was almost finished with my bachelor's degree as well. Before I realized it, she was elevated to higher positions and now she is like my boss. I was shocked! She didn't have the experience as me and just a brand-new graduate herself, plus I had to train her. I was very depressed about it and suddenly understood what workplace discrimination could be like. I weathered the storm there until I graduated from college. But by graduation, I was diagnosed with lupus. Eventually I quit my job and moved to Atlanta to be around family for support. As I was dealing with lupus alone with Leeann in Tallahassee and I was uncomfortable.

While I was living in Tallahassee, I dated a Nigerian man for several years. My family and friends knew him. We were almost like an item. I mean we spent lots of time with each other. We travelled together and he wined and dined me many times. By far, this was one of my most enjoyable relationships ever. All of a sudden, he went to Nigeria for a holiday and came back married. He claimed that a wife was chosen for him and he had to get married according to his tradition. I was hurt and torn apart but I eventually moved on. I said to myself that he is not indispensable! We are still friends and we share fun memories. To say the least some of my best dating times in this life has been with him.

A blunder in my life that I really despise and don't even like to think of is my second marriage! He was a pig! He won the record for abuse spouse in my books! I shouldn't have married him. He had all the "no signs" but I overlooked all of them. I will tell you this for fact that by far he was the most sexually appealing and best lovemaking man I have ever encountered. Maybe that kept me attracted to him! In retrospect, this is why he has many women, with many children. Sometimes I feel like he was a sperm donor. Thankfully I didn't make his statistics. During my marriage to him, he had several affairs and even fathered other children. He was a gigolo! Women spend money on him and buy his love. I didn't know what I was thinking but he got me like all his other women. One thing that got me convinced that he was a changed man was when he quit smoking. He went cold turkey with smoking and I was impressed. His lovemaking even got better. But after a while of dealing with his promiscuity and scared of my life for sexually transmitted diseases, I decided to divorce him. I didn't want to because it was my second marriage and I wanted it to work. I was afraid of the stigma that is associated with having more than one marriage. My lupus went crazy in my body and I was in and out of the hospital. I made up my mind to leave him. My life is better than stupid sex, which I have managed to experience some better ones after him.

Whenever I think about lupus and why lupus came upon me, I think about many possibilities that would have brought on this evil. I am certain that most of the scenarios I have written about have some level of contribution to bringing on the monster lupus in my life. Thankfully, I never smoked, did drugs, or excessive drinking of alcohol. If I had engaged in any of these, they would have caused more detriments to my situation. Especially smoking! With my interstitial lung disease, smoke in my lungs would have surely killed me soonest! My doctor even told me that had I smoked, my situation would have been worse. So I am thankful that I did not engage in such activities. I have come a long way in life and have overcome many obstacles. In this light, I see lupus as another obstacle course in my life and I shall overcome!

5

Choosing Me!

With this being my final chapter of my dear lupus and me, as well as how I am winning my battles, I wanted to give some survival tactics that I have engaged in my life that has brought me this far. Maybe it would be beneficial to my fellow lupus sufferers or folks who are walking in similar shoes as mine or an eye-opener to the world. I would like to discuss how I survived childhood pressures with sexual harassment, emotional turmoil, physical abuse, early marriage, marital abuse, workplace discrimination, and lupus' ups and downs.

Surviving childhood abuse in Sierra Leone was not easy because adults or people with money and/or power are always correct. If a young girl or boy says the old man or woman put his or her hands in my underwear, the first thing the community will be inclined to say is that that child is lying. Additionally, older people who do these acts threaten younger people and sometimes bribe them over-time. They put the fear in young people and because the fear that bad may come out if they tell, they never speak of it. Because I fear of what the outcome would be, I just tend to forget like it never happened. So when I was sexually molested, I just ran away and never go near that individual or stay alone with them. I remembered when I was about thirteen years old, I went for a vacation to Bo, a city away from Freetown to visit a kind and favorite uncle of mine. He lived in a one-bedroom and living room space. He slept in his room by himself and I was to sleep in the living room. But I was uncomfortable to spend the night in the living room. I am always afraid alone. There was a young girl, my age that lived in the same compound so I thought I would sleep with her. She lived with her sister and husband along with their kids.

71

At bedtime, her room door opened and the brother-in-law appeared. He had sex with the girl for a very long time and it seems the poor girl was exhausted. He turned her every way that he wanted! After watching them I felt bad for the girl as she looked wiped out and he had the biggest penis ever! When he finished, he came to me and wanted to have sex with me as well. I resisted and fought back. It was a rough night and I couldn't wait for the morning. I cut my holidays short and went back to Freetown the next day. I don't think I ever mentioned this event to anyone ever. I just think they wouldn't believe me. I am sure that the abuse continued with that young girl. I never followed up with her and I had no interest to visit that compound henceforth. There were many other sexual abuses that were close to happening to me and I managed to escape! When I was younger, I thought it was normal for older men to do this with younger people as I experienced it many times. As I grow older, I started to learn that I could resist and fight back and that is what I did. I really didn't have that person to discuss these events with. This is the case for so many young people in Sierra Leone at that time and it includes boys and girls as well. We keep these experiences in the back of our brains and never think about them. Also, my very own half-brother sexually molested me as well. I tried to block this in my mind and never spoke about it. I had the nerve to share it with some members of my family. They found it hard to believe and they questioned me too. They wanted to know why didn't I tell. That's how the story goes for these and it just died down. Many of these stories are real and it happens a lot in Sierra Leone.

As grown-ups, talking to some of my close relatives and friends, boys and girls, I found that a great many of them have suffered sexual abuses as well. Most of the time, the abuses come from older and respectable people in the community or household, which may include close family members. One of my older male friends from Sierra Leone told me a sad story that he was molested around age six or seven by his older cousin. His cousin was in high school or so and visited them during the long holidays. My friend's parent allowed the older cousin to spend the nights with my friend who was about seven years old at the time. He confides in me that his cousin would penetrate his rear end with his penis. It hurts and he cried and fought back. But the cousin convinced him that it was OK and if he tells his parents, he would be in big trouble. He frightened him and as a young boy, he fell for it. He said one night, he was so hard on him that he screamed and his mom ran to the room but the cousin lied and handled the situation like all was good. Then the cousin told him that he saved the situation as my friend would have been in a big trouble.

I know that the case of sexual abuse happens a lot to young people in Sierra Leone but I don't really know the extent of it. One reason is due to communal living. Cousins and extended family live together. Sometimes nonrelatives are rented sections of a family house and they live there over a period of time. My house I grew up in was very similar. There were a few pedophilias living in my house and abused many young girls and boys including myself. Our parents never knew about it. Some people knew but kept quiet. As children, we didn't know how to begin to discuss these issues. So we shared them by bed-wetting, afraid of the dark, or being alone. Sadly, most of us were never rescued! I think a huge population of girls and boys may be victims. It may be worth a research! Young people are scared and they are gullible with experience like this at times. We must increase education in this area.

I made sure that I always protect my little ones, especially my daughter from such devastation. I rarely allow Leeann for sleepovers except if I am comfortable with the family and I always question her about her experience with any sleepovers and playtimes. When I see or suspect sexual and/or emotional abuses, I am quick to bring it out and save the victim. Although my actions to be quiet about the abuses then were not the best decision, but given the fact that no one would hear or listen, I thought silence was the right thing at that time. Maybe my mom and my sisters would have stood up for me if I had told them but I wasn't sure of them or how they would take it. We didn't have such discussions at home. If it were today, I may have reported to the police or get help. Things are much better about how they handle these incidences nowadays in Sierra Leone and the world at large. More information is provided to young people to report and people are speaking out for them nowadays. I want to encourage young people who are suffering from such abuses to report it or get help. Storing these abuses in my brain from childhood may have caused some overload on my mind, body, and soul that I became weak causing my immune system be broken down. Some of these effects may have allowed lupus to enter my body. So if you are a victim of any abuse, please report it or find a way to off-load it out of your system and mind. Always remember you are never alone. As an adult now, I don't take bullshit from anyone. I set a line of demarcation for myself. Please get help!

For physical and mental abuses, I often run away from the environment or just stay away. Case in point, when I was living with the old lady at Kissy, I ran away due to nonstop mental, physical, and emotional abuses. The only abuse that I regret subduing myself into is FGM! I feel that pain up till now and I only wish I had run away here too. Really, I wasn't aware of exactly what was going on in the FGM society. If only I had the slightest clue, I would flee faster than lighting and seek help somewhere. After my most painful experience with FGM, I vouched that I will never condone it! Especially when my baby sister was mutilated right in front of my eyes and I couldn't help her! I promised to save all my little sisters and girls from the traumas of FGM. When one finds himself or herself in a situation where you can flee, please do so and you will be doing your body a whole lot of good and saving yourself from stress and diseases in the long run.

Although I often flee from abuses, they still stay in my mind. I prayed a lot as a child. I spent many times praying for God to end my pains. I also enjoyed doing schoolwork. I had a feeling that education would make a difference in my life one day. So I gave school my uttermost strength and courage. Also, I enjoyed writing. So I had pen pals from all over the world. I write and ask them about kid's lives in their different countries and they would tell me their stories. I was very connected to my pen pals until the post office system broke down and I traveled to the United States. I got involved in prayers, schoolwork, and writing to pen pals to escape my misery. I also enjoyed hair braiding. It seems to me that I braided all my problems and stresses on doing different styles of braids for my friends and family members. Up till now, I enjoy hair braiding as a source of relief of my mental problems. It is somewhat therapeutic and sometimes I make money from it as well.

In my days, after high school, it seems young girls often get married. I had many of my friends who got married before me. So I thought marriage was the right thing to do. The man I married was about twelve years older than me. I looked up to him as a big brother and I respected him too. He was very studious and hardworking. My older sisters knew him in college and they liked him very much. They thought he would be a good partner for me. I had a boyfriend that I loved at the time. However, he was abroad studying and I hard he had other girlfriends. So I decided to forget about him. The man I married threatened me to forget about him or there will be consequences. So I just turned my mind off the boyfriend I loved for peace sake. Also, I respect my sisters' suggestions. I thought that listening to my sisters to have a relationship with the man I married would be better for me. Come to find out, he was possessive, controlling, and sometimes he hurts me physically as well as mentally. I tried running away from him several times but he always plead and promise not to do it again. Eventually, I just decided to stick around with him and hope for better days. He was coming to the United States to study and we got married in the hope that I would join him as his wife. Long story short, we moved to America together in 1983 at my tender age of eighteen years old. The physical, mental, and emotional abuses continued. Sometimes, I will react at him and fight back as well.

One time, I caught him cheating. I was very upset and it blew my mind away. We were always arguing or fighting over one thing or another. It was very difficult during these times. The police were involved. The university was involved as well. We were forced to get counseling. I didn't even know what counseling was all about. But I was willing to try it to save our marriage. Once, we left the marriage counseling mad. As soon as we were out of the building, we got into a big fight in the parking lot. The FSU police had to break us up apart. I was tired and just fed up. I ran away again. We actually got divorced. After about six months away, he found me and he apologized. For my daughter's sake and the fact that I really wanted to give our marriage a chance, I came back. However, it did not last too long and the abuses continued. So one day I moved out and found my own apartment in Tallahassee. This was the end of us. After about ten plus years of ups and downs, it was suddenly over. Right after these many ups and downs with my marriage, I began to feel ill. Sometimes, I would just pass out for no reason. Then I would wake up suddenly like nothing happened. My daughter and my niece, Dr. Fatu Forna Sesay, who lived with me were concerned and scared at times. It happened a lot and then I started undergoing medical tests to find out the problems. I started to notice strange health patterns but I didn't take it serious!

Later, I dated a Nigerian in Tallahassee. It was by far my best relationship while it lasted. Although he ended up disappointing me and married someone else, I had the best dating experience with him. When we were dating, we shared good times together. I had other dates in between as well. But my relationship with the Nigerian lasted a while and longer than any of my other relationships. Then I dated another Sierra Leonean, whom I ended marrying for my second marriage. *It* was the worse relationship ever! He was abusive—emotionally, physically, and mentally. By far my worse choice ever! Leaving both relationships were difficult. Especially my second husband for fear of a failed second marriage and the stigma that is associated with it. However, trying to survive these relationships took a toll on my lupus. I had bouts with lupus and relapses. In fact, this is how my lungs started to come into play with lupus. All of a sudden, something hit my mind and I woke up! I decided that I must let these relationships out of my life. So I did and life goes on! It was a decision that I had to make, especially for the later relationship as lupus was having a party in my life and I had to break the party up. Disconnecting from these relationships were the way forward for me and a very positive move for my life.

Before I got diagnosed with lupus, I worked for the State Government of Florida for more than ten years. I build up my professionalism working in these offices. Later, I worked for Emory

University, Georgetown University, and the University of Sierra Leone. Additionally, I have engaged my time with consultancies all over the world as well. I have always enjoyed my work environments. Every workplace may pose its ups and downs but I try to get the best out of it. I learned team playing and tactfulness are some of the keys to survive in a workplace. Of course, one's knowledge of his or her duties and responsibilities for one's job are paramount. I received recognitions in my jobs always. For the most part, I get along well with my colleagues. However, there was a case in Tallahassee that shook the hell out of me and for the first time I experienced workplace discrimination. It bothered me a whole lot. I thought I could handle it but it got to me badly. Sadly, it was around the same time I was diagnosed with lupus. I got very ill and had to take six months of sick leave. Although it was sick leave, I used the opportunity to finish up my degree and participated on a study abroad program in France. I tried to relax a whole lot and just enjoyed the moment. It was even more fun when Leeann came along and we spent some valuable time together with my best friend Abi Banya. I returned back to work after six months. I graduated the following year in May 2001. After graduation, I packed my stuff and relocated to Atlanta right away. This way we would be near family should I need assistance dealing with lupus. After about fifteen years of living in Tallahassee, I closed that chapter in my life. It was a huge change! Again with God by my side and family support we pulled through it.

I narrated all this because learning to deal with these crises in my life got me better ready to handle the real lupus. These events were traumatic and life changing, but the changes and adaptations for lupus are unmeasurable. For instance, when I have a lupus crisis, one couldn't tell by looking at me. In the beginning, I was confused myself. Some days, I am well and some days I am in a lot of pain. It could be so painful I could hardly walk. I moved slowly. People constantly judge me. They look at me and assume I am so slow and they walk past me. I cried silently in pain and in disbelief as to the way my life is today. Before lupus in my life, I would run down ten flights of stairs and even ran long races. Now, I have to wait for the elevators. Older folks and handicap people will want to push me out of the way assuming that I am well and I could take the stairs. I often smile and let them use the elevators as I waited for the next elevator. Due to my health issues, the doctor had given me a note to let my job adjust my work hours as well. So I was able to use flex time. This means that I could work from my home or come into work early and leave later. Moving forward, I learned to give myself more than enough time and make sure I leave before anyone else to be on time. But when I am late or needed the extra time, people are very accommodative.

While I was in college for both undergraduate and graduate programs, I always utilize the students with disability office as they have a wealth of information and ways to contribute to the lives of the physically challenged people and make things easier for us. For instance, my arms get cold and painful during exams. Sometimes the temperatures in the classroom could slow you down as well. At the physically challenge offices for students, they provide special rooms with temperature adjustments, time and half for exams if you need it, bigger prints for people with sight issues, special equipment to aid the deaf, comfortable chairs and sometimes snacks for us. I made sure I utilized the assistance as much as possible. Often, they would provide financial aids in grants to assist with our school expenses as well.

Also, I have serious challenges with using the bathrooms, I often have to use the handicap stalls as I need to hold on to the rails when I used the bathrooms. I remembered one time, a physically challenged person, who was on crutches yelled at me for using the handicap stalls. I was quiet and waited until she came out of the bathroom. Then I nicely told her that all handicap situations are not visible. I told her that I just wanted her to know that I needed to use that stall and that's why I used it. I do have a disability that is not visible. She was shocked and apologized. Slowly, I learned to speak up for myself as I continue to learn the loops along with the challenges of living with lupus. I quickly learned to be my own advocate. Also, when I need help, I asked for it and most of the time people do help me.

The longer I live with lupus, the more I learned to understand it and learn to advocate for my well-being. With lupus you are giving so many medications. They try to see if the medications will work for you. A medication that is constant for most lupus and immune diseases is prednisone. When there is a lupus flare, the first thing they want to do is increase prednisone. Prednisone helps but it blows you up like a balloon and sometimes brings about other complications. One time, I was very ill and I had a relapse. Before I realized it I was on 60 mg of prednisone. I took the dosage for about a week. I blew up so bad and gained thirty pounds in no time. Before you know it my sugar went up, my pressure rose, and my heart was constantly racing. Since that episode, whenever I get to the hospital, I negotiate with them regarding the amount of prednisone I am given. Usually the doctors work with me on the dose. As soon as I get out of the hospital, I worked hard and lose the weight and my medical issues subsided. I learned that one has to be involved with your health issues and advocate for your health. It's your life and no one could fight for it better than you. Moving forward, I decided to discuss my health needs which include medications as well. I am very hands-on, when it comes to my health.

Another time, I was very ill and my daughter and son-in-law called the ambulance to pick me up. I knew they would prefer to take me to the nearest hospital but I prefer Mount Sinai since my medical team is affiliated with that hospital. I negotiated with them to take me to Mount Sinai by informing them that my medical team are located at Mount Sinai and I will be at proximity to them if I am at that hospital. They listened to me and took me to Mount Sinai.

Another crisis area for me is dealing with the oxygen tank. Since my lungs have gotten weaker overtime, I had no choice but to walk around with a portable oxygen tank. I never like using oxygen. It made me feel like I am not a full human being and like I live an assisted living life! So I always fought against using it. But let me tell you, when push comes to pull, you pull! During my many hospital stays, when I could hardly breathe, the oxygen was my rescue. After hospital stays, I felt like I don't need them anymore. But when I walk up hills, climb stairs, very long walks and hastily doing something, running for the bus, pains shoot up my spine and I go into shortness of breath mode. Sometimes, I feel sad for myself. I just wouldn't carry the oxygen because of the fear I had and fearing of how people will judge me. One time, I was really feeling sick and I went to see my pulmonary doctor. He gave simple tests to check my oxygen when walking. It dropped fast and low so quick, he stopped and said you need oxygen! He said, "You need to use oxygen regularly!" He said it's, "Very serious!" He told me that there could be serious consequences that may prove fatal if I don't use it more often. He was very serious and so were my other medical doctors in my team. Finally, I decided to carry it around. First thing I did was to find a vendor that would service me a smaller and portable tank, which I did. Then I made up my mind to care less about what people say or think about people carrying the oxygen tank. No kidding, one time I was walking and I heard people discussing about me and the oxygen that smoking will let you carry oxygen tanks. Truth is, I never smoked! Oh well, there we go again; I just kept on moving and thanking God for the opportunity that I have to use the oxygen tank. Now, I carry my tank with me everywhere I go. People stare at me, and sometimes people sympathize with me as well as lend me a helping hand when they see me and my oxygen tank. Sadly, there are times when I would take a break from wearing the oxygen and they would ignore me and assume I am perfectly well. So to get assistance, especially on a full bus or train ride, I put my oxygen on and people give me a seat or render a helping hand. Sometimes, when people don't offer me a seat or help, I asked them kindly and some gladly give me their seats or assistance, while others reluctantly do it. I am very friendly with my oxygen and I use it faithfully. It is helping my breathing a whole lot. Sometimes I place the oxygen in a bag while I move around. Other times, I carry it around in its sac. Wherever I go, it is me and my oxygen friend. My grandson, Malik, usually say don't judge me! So I put on my oxygen with a "don't judge me" attitude! In fact, I was thinking about doing some decorative colorful stuff to wrap around the cords of the tank. My daughter thought it was a great idea and we are working on it. Hey don't judge, it works for me!

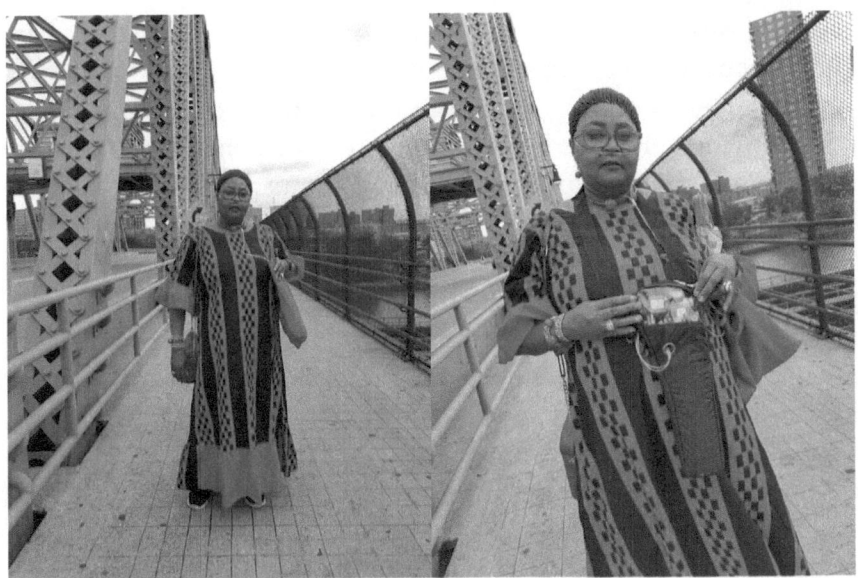

Oxygen tank in my bag   Oxygen out of the bag

Many a time, I have to adjust my life pattern to live with lupus. Just imagine having gone through higher education and up to master's level but couldn't really work in your field of expertise. It is heart rendering! I was hoping by now, in my age, I would have an awesome and enjoyable career, which I was on the path to doing, but lupus, why? You take over me sometimes! You make me weep sometimes!

I had to move to Sierra Leone in 2009 and I was enjoying work along with life. But due to lupus and Sierra Leone not able to accommodate my medical needs, I had to move back to the United States. I had to make the difficult decision of where to really settle down. I know that I didn't want to live alone. I have choices to live with many relatives and one particular friend/relative, Haoua Cullibally, would be an excellent choice. She lived with me in Florida and we got along very well. She said that I could live with her if I want to. But I chose to live with Leeann, my daughter and family, as Leeann highly recommends that I live with them. Due to the fact that she is a working wife and mother, it would be quite juggling between cities to see me when I am ill. So I thought living with them would be fine. Plus I enjoyed spending time with my grandson and Leeann as well.

I really wasn't sure how my son-in-law would fit in. But we lived in Sierra Leone for a bit and so I expect it to be OK.

So far, it is working out very well. They love and enjoy my cooking. My daughter also enjoyed getting her hair done by me and she saves money as well. I love and adore the company of Malik too! He brings me so much joy in my life. Now that I have a new grandbaby, Makeen Abdulai is even better and sweeter! For the most part we get along with each other. Once in a while we get on each other's nerve and I will take a break from them. It has been a huge adjustment living with them and I have to check myself many a time. Especially living with my son-in-law! His family dynamics and their nonacceptance of my daughter into their family have caused many commotions to the peaceful lives of them as a family. It bothers me as a mother to see my only daughter go through such drama of culture clash. I pray for God's guidance and protection for them all the time. One thing they have going for them and I admire about it of them is the love and patience for each other. I believe they survive because of their love for each other. I truly admire my daughter's courage and perseverance over the fact that her husband's parents rejects her so very much but she is still sticking with her husband! Our space is small like most New York City living and makes it even more complicated to live together. But we are working on getting a bigger place. To give a break from ourselves and our little space, I visit friends, families, go to Africa, or just do something to get away and travel. These mini vacations are really good to suppress my lupus as I free my mind of everything and just concentrate on me. It is a way to reduce my stress and rejuvenate my mind, body, and soul! Additionally, during these vacations, I go with my best friend Abi B and/or families along with other friends. We went to South Africa, Lesotho, Jamaica, England, and of course Sierra Leone. I have also been to Japan and the Bahamas. Here are some pictures of some of trips around the world with families and friends.

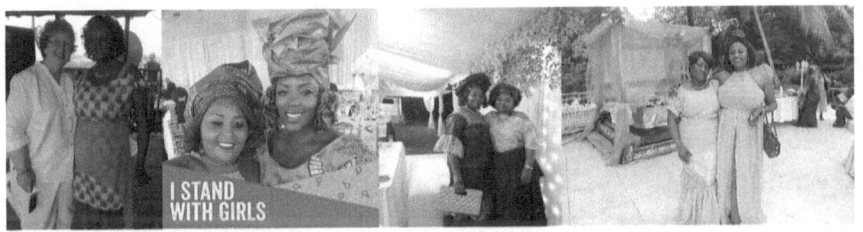

Julie and I, Freetown, Leeann and I, Florida Abi
and I, Jamaica Comfort and I, Freetown

Sometimes we do family outings and vacations together. They are very patient with me as I walk slower. They always have to wait for me. Also I use the bathrooms more than they do due to problems with incontinency. I think the medications made me use the bathrooms more as well. But also, I read that FGM and COPD could bring on incontinency. I have discussed these with an OBGYN/ Endocrinologist and we are working on how they could help me. But my family always let me ease myself whenever nature calls. I really appreciate them for caring and sharing with me. Living with them is not rosy all the time. After all, it's their house and I feel like I am invading sometimes. But my daughter constantly let me know that she is OK to share with me and her husband is OK too. Sometimes I feel a bit bullied by them when they are firm with me. Like when I was out of the hospital after about three months. My appetite was poor, and I was very picky about foods. So I wasted a lot of foods. One day my son-in-law said they would stop giving me food if I don't eat much. I couldn't just eat and I had no appetite and they thought I was been wasteful. But it's their house and I tried to do things their way so we can live in peace. I treasure my time with my grandchildren and my daughter as well as her husband. So I tried my best to weather the storm with them. I rather live with them than anyone else. So I try very hard so we can live in peace. When I feel that we need a break, I take a trip to visit friends and relatives. People judge that I shouldn't be staying with them. But I discussed it with them and they are very OK with me living with them. They told me to stop worrying about what people think and focus on my health. I am doing just this and it's all good. People stop judging!

Additionally, Leeann has Young Men's Christian Association (YMCA) family membership. I work out there a lot and I have made many friends there. When Leeann and my niece, Fatu were younger, I was a member of the YMCA and we enjoyed working out there. Now she enjoys it with her family. It's a great family work-out place. My grandson Malik is in karate and swimming. In fact, he is now an advance green belt. I do aquatic aerobics at the YMCA. I feel like the aquatic group is a team on its own. These are matured women and men who are all trying to keep fit and taking care of their health issues. Our instructors are awesome and we look forward to aquatic aerobics every morning.

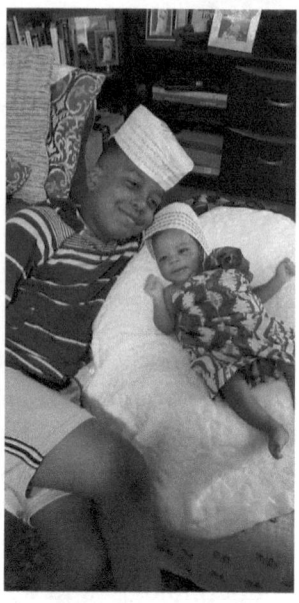

Malik and Makeen

Jon, one of the instructors is very good at his class, although they are all good but he leaps out of the way to ensure we are doing the right thing and tell us how to work out to make a difference.

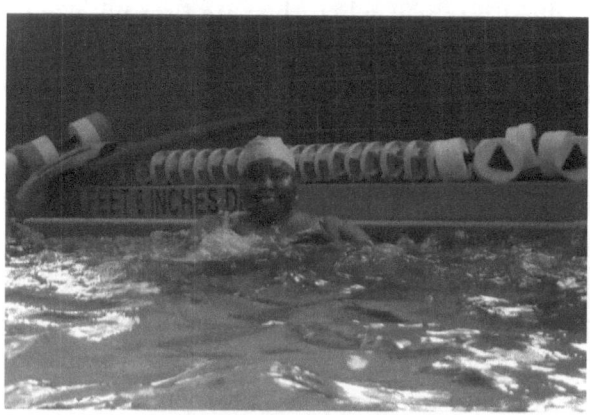

Enjoying Water Aerobics

"People drama" has caused some stress in my life and lupus relapses more than anything. This has direct link with family members and friends or people I interact with daily. For some reasons, I end up with losers and user-type friendships once in a while. In Sierra Leone, I learned that when some people come too close to you, you need to be awake otherwise you will be broken! One of my sisters, who we constantly get on each other's nerve more often than my other sisters, recommended a driver to drive me around Freetown. Freetown is a small city with rough and untrained drivers. Most of the drivers could not read and often do not understand road signs. One needs a driver to drive one around sometimes. Anyhow, I got the driver and he drove me for about six months and ended up stealing about ten thousand dollars from me. This was money that was to be used for USL events. The stealing caused lots of professional problems for me at USL. Up till now, I have never set eyes on that driver and my sister hasn't heard or seen him either.

There was another young girl who, claimed I was her mother/ friend. I was very kind to her and assisted her with many situations. She ended up stealing money from me and almost destroyed my relationship between one of my sisters. Also, family ups and downs were a bit bothersome at times. Stressful events, like the death of my mother; dealing with the many trials and tribulations in the marriage of my daughter, which is a book in the making; dealing with family members "wahala"(drama-krio word); and many other fracases in life are quite stressful as well. It seems like stressful events find me and somehow, I manage to loop myself into them. With lupus in my life, learning to eliminate stress is very important. By the grace of God and with lots of prayers, I was able to make a comeback from the overbearingness of these situations. Now, I try hard not be bothered by anyone or circumstances. When I feel it's too much, I move away and/or engage my mind into something else. I am using the same tactic in dealing with families, friends and/or circumstances I face nowadays. No more stress from anyone or any circumstances, as these exacerbate my lupus crises.

To really help me manage my stresses better, I have engaged in mental health therapy and physical activities as well. I have a mental counselor I meet with once a week to discuss the way forward and plan to keep myself engaged. She hears and listens to all my worries and has a way to take them away. She comes from a neutral perspective and talks to me in a layman's term. I don't know what life would be without her in my journey this far. She is amazing! I really would suggest mental therapy when you know you need it. If you are not sure, just try it. If you have situations in life that is above and beyond you, engage mental therapy. God is great, but in addition to our faith, we need solid talks and connection on earth. Mental therapy could be it!

Also, my daughter and family, some of my friends, especially Abi Banya, Dr. Julia Goodwin, Haoua Cullibally, and a few others have been a blessing and my source for laughter, joy, and peace. My family members and extended families have been awesome in keeping my head and mind in check. My mother was my rock but since she is in heaven, I look upon her as my guiding angel. Really cannot imagine what my journey with lupus would have been hadn't I have these folks in my life. I thank God for them each and every day. I exercise faithfully! I do water aerobics at the Harlem YMCA five times a week, plus some exercises in the gymnasium as well. My aqua aerobics team and the YMCA have been a strong outlet for me too. Going there and just exercising and hanging out with very brave and strong women have just rejuvenated my soul. Please find positive people in your life and hang with them, it is worth your living. Additionally, I set a walking goal of ten thousand steps a day. I meet the goals sometimes but I get to a minimum of five thousand steps per day. The only time that I cannot make at least five thousand steps is when I feel sick. I usually take a few days off from YMCA and walking. Exercises and mental relaxation have helped me a great deal.

Finally, my God is more than awesome to me and has favored me highly! I get so sick, weak, and hopeless at times. But I bounce back! Sometimes I can't believe myself. Even my doctors are amazed. They often say my spirit is why I am living! My catholic faith continues to take me along each and every day. I mean, I have about 25 percent scarring of my lungs and still function OK, especially with my friend, the oxygen! I feel like God chose my medical team from day one. From Tallahassee Memorial Hospital, to Grady and Gwinnet Hospitals in Atlanta, to Holy Cross Hospital and Washington Hospital Center in

Maryland and Washington, DC, to Mekene Hospital in Dallas, to Choithram, St. Josephs and Connaught Hospitals in Freetown and the great Mount Sinai in New York City are been chosen by his grace to have brought me this far. I am feeling much better each day and I continue to pray for miracles as I would like to spend more quality life with families and friends and especially my grandchildren. To God be the glory!

Lola, congratulations on the publication of your first book! It is an unbelievable story of strength over adversity, courage over fear and determination by a young African woman in a strange, different culture. Your book is inspiring. I recommend it as a text to colleges preparing students in the fields of psychology, sociology, social work, and education and health. I wish you success with your book, good health and long life.

-Julia Goodwin, Ph.D. Mentor and Friend

This is a powerful book that people must read. I am so sorry that you had to go through so much pain and suffering. You have overcome so much, and you are truly amazing. I am so lucky to have gotten to know you.

-Martha Morgan, Mental Therapist

Lola Aforo has privileged us with a glimpse into her tumultuous life experiences. In Lupus or Me? I Chose Me! she imparts a story that illustrates why women everywhere must have guaranteed societal support in every country. Her memoir, brief but important, shows how women are often marginalized in society through their personal experiences, most especially in marriage. She writes with a dignified simplicity that speaks to some of the most urgent needs based on gender and race. This is a book written by a courageous woman who faced every adversity with hope. I read it through in two days and feel blessed to have Lola as a sister friend and to confirm what I already knew that she is a decent, moral, steadfast human being.

-Dr. Elain Terry, Mathematics Professor and Mentor

Lola, thanks for giving me the opportunity to read your book. It is really an awesome piece. It is a realistic account of your battles with Lupus. Before Lupus, I knew you had a hard time in the US upon arrival, but I never realized the extent of your problems.

Now I have renewed admiration for you! I hope other patients of lupus will benefit from your book. I wish you success with it.

-Mrs. Ebun Strasser-King Aforo, Lawyer and my big sister

The author is very pragmatic, brave and plain straight-forward in describing her practical traumatic life events with cultural taboos. The advice and counsel to victims of sexual abuse, FGM and Lupus by this strong-willed, resilient super Advocate is both valuable and beneficial to young innocent African children, their parents/guardians as well as worldwide advocacy officials. From start to finish, I could not put down this very inspirational book. Bravo and proud of you, Lola Aforo, one of my best friends and colleague who used her strong personality and honesty to face the evil causes of Lupus disease and her brave strategies of dealing with for decades of her life. A highly intellectual, academic and global community advocate deserves a "Best Seller" ranking. I recommend this author for empirical research studies on the topics of "Lupus", "Sexual Abuse" as well as "FGM". The book is also an excellent read during this global pandemic shutdown. I thoroughly enjoyed it.

-Dr. Lauretta Will Sillah, CEO, People's
Foundation for Humanity Development

At a time like this when Sierra Leone is forced to confront rising levels of sexual based violence, this book is a must read for anyone interested in understanding the myriad of challenges faced by women and girls in Sierra Leone.

Lola Aforo is a gifted writer. Her frankness, courage and easygoing writing style makes this book more than her battle with lupus. It is also a testament to the power of faith, love and the endless endurance of the human spirit. I highly recommend it.

-Alimamy Koroma, Lawyer and Mentee

About the Author

Lola Aforo is a native of Sierra Leone who currently lives in Harlem, New York City. She completed her undergraduate education at Florida State University and her postgraduate at Georgetown University in Washington DC. Ms. Aforo has a passion for public speaking and youth empowerment programs. Also, she is interested in writing and telling stories about Sierra Leone and USA. She engages in educational projects, youth development, and empowerment programs in New York City. Ms. Aforo is involved in many charitable organizations in Sierra Leone. She currently leads on a feeding project in Sierra Leone, which is named after her late mother called "Si Jemi Kitchen". *Lupus or Me? I Chose Me!* is her very first published novel. She plans to write some more novels in the future. She has a daughter, son-in-law, and two grandchildren.